DEDICATION

To my terrific grandchildren,
Ni-zhoni and Simon.
—MLW

To my loving parents,
my wonderful wife,
and my awesome children.
—HS

ACKNOWLEDGMENT

I would like to acknowledge Melanie Nelson, PhD, for helping me with the list of parenting books and training programs.

—MLW

I acknowledge the aid of Arthur Robin, PhD, for help in the identification of certain rating scales.

—HS

Clinical Diagnosis and Management of Attention-Deficit/Hyperactivity Disorder (ADHD)

First Edition

Mark L. Wolraich, MD
Director of Child Study Center
CMRI/Shaun Walters Professor of Pediatrics
Oklahoma University Health Sciences Center

Howard Schubiner, MD
Department of Internal Medicine,
Providence Hospital and Medical Centers,
St John Health
Clinical Professor, Wayne State University

PROFESSIONAL
COMMUNICATIONS, INC.

Professional Communications, Inc.
A Medical Publishing Company

Marketing Office:
400 Center Bay Drive
West Islip, NY 11795
(t) 631/661-2852
(f) 631/661-2167

Editorial Office:
PO Box 10
Caddo, OK 74729-0010
(t) 580/367-9838
(f) 580/367-9989

For orders only, please call
1-800-337-9838
or visit our website at
www.pcibooks.com

ISBN: 978-1-932610-39-0

Printed in the United States of America

DISCLAIMER

The opinions expressed in this publication reflect those of the authors. However, the authors make no warranty regarding the contents of the publication. The protocols described herein are general and may not apply to a specific patient. Any product mentioned in this publication should be taken in accordance with the prescribing information provided by the manufacturer.

This text is printed on recycled paper.

TABLE OF CONTENTS

Introduction and History	1
Etiology, Prevalence, and Long-Term Outcomes	2
Diagnosis of ADHD	3
Treating ADHD as a Chronic Illness	4
Medication Treatment	5
Psychosocial Treatments	6
Alternative Treatments	7
Substance Abuse Disorders and Issues Related to ADHD	8
Appendix	9
Abbreviations/Acronyms	10
Index	11

TABLES

Table 3.1 Core Symptoms of ADHD 24

Table 3.2 Evaluating Reporter Disagreement of ADHD Symptoms in Children 27

Table 3.3 Other Criteria Required for the Diagnosis of ADHD 27

Table 3.4 *DSM-IV*–Based ADHD Rating Scales for Children and Adolescents 30

Table 3.5 *DSM-IV*–Based Rating Scales for Adults 32

Table 3.6 *DSM-IV* Criteria for Oppositional Defiant Disorder 36

Table 3.7 *DSM-IV* Criteria for Conduct Disorder 37

Table 3.8 *DSM-IV* Criteria for Major Depressive Episode 38

Table 3.9 *DSM-IV* Criteria for Manic Episode 38

Table 4.1 Elements of a Chronic-Illness Approach to Treatment 46

Table 4.2 Questions Pertaining to the Post–High School Adolescent With ADHD 53

Table 5.1 Stimulant Medications: Dosing and Pharmacokinetics 66

Table 5.2 Proportion of Responders and Nonresponders to DEX and MPH 67

Table 5.3 Proportion of Nonresponders to One Stimulant Who Responded to the Other Stimulant 68

Table 6.1 Books and Web Resources Recommended for Parent Training 100

Table 6.2 Parenting Programs 101

Table 6.3 Principal Elements of Parent Training 104

Table 6.4 Daily Report Card 108

Table 8.1 Levels of Substance Use and Abuse and Suggested Management Approaches 126

Table 8.2 Precautions to Avoid Abuse of Stimulants and Red Flags for Misuse or Diversion 128

FIGURES

Figure 1.1 Attention-Deficit/Hyperactivity Disorder Timeline....11

Figure 2.1 Percentage of Patients Meeting ADHD Core Symptom Requirements in Epidemiologic Studies (1994)....18

Figure 3.1 ADHD Diagnostic Algorithm for Children and Adolescents....25

Figure 3.2 ADHD Diagnostic Algorithm for Adults....26

Figure 4.1 ADHD Management Plan....48

Figure 5.1 Blood Concentration of Methylphenidate Over Time....60

Figure 5.2 Methylphenidate Dose Response: Efficacy From Crossover Phase Indicating Improvement in ADHD Symptoms With Increased Dose....61

Figure 5.3 Effect of Metadate CD and Placebo on CTGI Scores in Children and Adolescents Treated in a Community Classroom Setting....70

Figure 5.4 Mean Changes From Baseline in CADS-P Total and Subscale Scores After 2-Weeks' Treatment With Ritalin LA or Placebo....71

Figure 5.5 Teacher IOWA Conners I/O Scores in Children With ADHD Treated With OROS MPH, IR MPH, or Placebo....72

Figure 5.6 Change in *DSM-IV* Symptom Clusters After 6-Weeks' Treatment With OROS Methylphenidate in Adults With ADHD....73

Figure 5.7 Adjusted Mean Changes From Predose in SKAMP Combined Scores in Children With ADHD Using Extended-Release Dexmethylphenidate, Extended-Release *d,l*-methylphenidate, or Placebo....74

Figure 5.8 Mean SKAMP-D Subscale Scores by Time Point in Children Age 6 to 12 Years With ADHD: Methylphenidate Transdermal System vs Placebo....75

Figure 5.9 Duration of Action of Methylphenidate Products....77

Figure 5.10 Duration of Action of Amphetamine Products 80

Figure 5.11 Percentage of Patients Improved vs Not Improved at Study End Point: Mixed Amphetamine Salts Extended-Release vs Placebo 82

Figure 5.12 Time-Course Changes in SKAMP and PERMP Scores Across Assessment Day in School-Age Children in a Laboratory Classroom Setting: Lisdexamfetamine Dimesylate, Mixed Amphetamine Salts Extended-Release, and Placebo 84

Figure 5.13 Change From Baseline in ADHD-RS Total Scores at Each Week in Patients Taking Lisdexamfetamine vs Placebo: ITT Population 87

Figure 5.14 Mean ADHD-RS-IV Total Scores for Adolescents Over 2 Years' Treatment With Atomoxetine 88

Figure 5.15 Medication Algorithm for Preschool-Age Patients 92

Figure 5.16 Medication Algorithm for Primary School-Age Through Adult Patients 93

Figure 8.1 Algorithm for Assessment and Treatment of Substance Abuse 123

APPENDICES

Appendix 1 Vanderbilt Parent-Assessment Scale 134

Appendix 2 Vanderbilt Parent-Assessment Follow-Up 138

Appendix 3 Vanderbilt Teacher-Asssessment Scale 140

Appendix 4 Vanderbilt Teacher-Assessment Follow-Up 144

Appendix 5 Pittsburgh Side-Effects–Rating Scale 146

1 Introduction and History

Attention-deficit/hyperactivity disorder (ADHD) is a common neurobiologic condition that has been clearly shown to have a significant impact on individuals who have the condition.[1] There has been more research undertaken on this condition than on any other mental disorder diagnosis in childhood and more than for many physical conditions. It has also become clear that it is not just a condition of childhood. The impairments caused by ADHD continue into adulthood and continue to require treatment for many of those individuals who have it.[2] Despite the research that documents these facts, ADHD continues to be a controversial disorder. There are many myths and much misinformation about the condition, as well as challenges in providing optimal treatment. The purpose of this book is to correct those myths and misinformation and to present the evidence about the condition in a practical framework so that clinicians can provide the best care possible for their patients with ADHD.

The following are corrections to some of the most common myths about ADHD:

- *It is not a newly created condition.* ADHD actually has a long history, although because of frequent name changes, it has appeared to have been discovered recently. Even though the condition was first introduced into the medical field around the turn of the century, a physician in the mid-19th century who wrote stories for children first described what have been the two behavioral dimensions of ADHD. Heinrich Hoffman, a German physician, described these dimensions via the two characters in a children's book, *Johnny Look-in-the-Air*, representing an inattentive easily distracted child (http://www.fln.vcu.edu/struwwel/guck_e.html. Accessed March 30, 2009) and *Fidgety Phil*, representing a hyperactive child (http://www.fln.vcu.edu/struwwel/philipp_e.html. Accessed March 30, 2009).[3] Both children were characterized as misbehaving children who suffered justified consequences. The sentiment that children with these characteristics are willfully misbehaving and deserve appropriate punishments remains a prominent sentiment among those who are skeptical about the condition.

The introduction of ADHD into the medical field came in 1902, at a meeting of the Royal College of Physicians when George Still described a disease he considered to be due to a defect in moral character (**Figure 1.1**).[4] He noted that the problem resulted in a child's inability to internalize rules and limits, and was manifest in patterns of restless, inattentive, and overaroused behaviors; thus he clearly described the core symptoms of inattention, hyperactivity, and impulsivity. Dr. Still suggested that children with the condition had likely experienced brain damage, but that the behavior could also arise from hereditary and environmental factors.

- *Most cases of ADHD are not due to brain damage.* The belief that brain damage was the major cause of the condition became more prominent after the 1917 to 1918 worldwide epidemic of influenza because common residual effects of influenza encephalitis in children were symptoms of restlessness, inattention, impulsivity, easy arousability, and hyperactivity.[5] However, there appeared to be a number of children with less-severe restlessness and no clear history of brain damage who, due to their behavior, still appeared to be impaired. This group of children was categorized in the 1960s as having a condition defined as minimal cerebral/brain dysfunction/damage (MBD). A prominent characteristic of this condition was what was described as soft neurologic signs. Soft neurologic signs are developmentally based signs such as the persistence of overflow activity beyond 9 years of age or continuing right-left confusion.

However, the lack of a relationship between brain damage and the condition caused concerns about the diagnostic label of MBD. Subsequent diagnos-

FIGURE 1.1 — Attention-Deficit/Hyperactivity Disorder Timeline

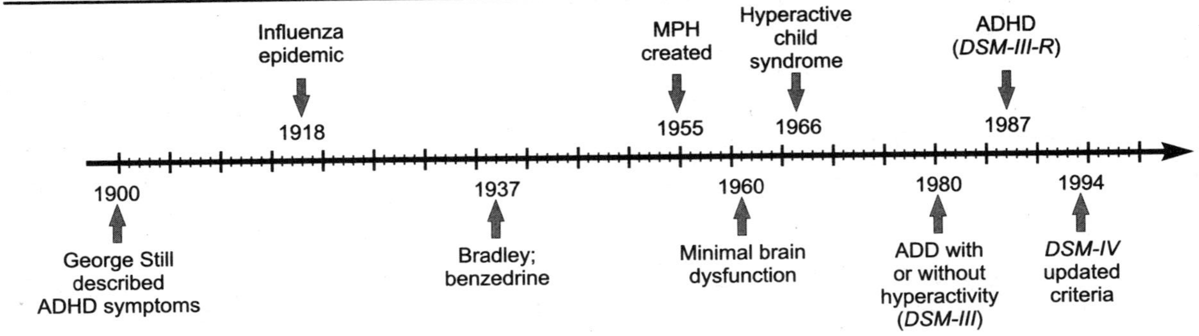

1

tic labels shifted to more behaviorally descriptive terms. These diagnostic names initially focused on the hyperactive behavior, including hyperkinetic impulse reaction disorder in the psychiatric classification system (*DSM-II*) and hyperactive child syndrome in the pediatric literature.

- *Hyperactivity is not the primary debilitating problem.* In 1980, the work of Virginia Douglas and others demonstrated that the predominantly debilitating aspect of ADHD is the inattention.[6] This finding shifted the focus from considering hyperactivity as the primary problem to considering inattention as the primary deficit. The revision of the diagnostic label to attention-deficit disorder (ADD) first occurred in 1980 with the revision of the American psychiatric diagnostic system (the *Diagnostic and Statistical Manual of Mental Disorders* to *DSM-III*).[7] This revision defined the three core behavioral dimensions of inattention, impulsivity, and hyperactivity. These core dimensions have remained constant in the subsequent diagnostic criteria, with the exception that hyperactivity and impulsivity have appeared to form one dimension in subsequent studies. The revision also defined two subtypes, ADD with and without hyperactivity.[8] Subsequently, the subtypes were eliminated in *DSM-IIIR*[9] and then because of better evidence redefined in *DSM-IV*[10] to the current subtypes of predominantly inattentive, predominantly hyperactive/impulsive, and combined subtypes.
- *ADHD can occur in girls.* While ADHD is more common in males, with a 3-4 to 1 ratio, it does occur quite frequently in females.[11] They are less like to exhibit hyperactivity and tend to be identified at an older age.
- *ADHD is not just a children's disorder that disappears by puberty.* In actuality, a majority of children with ADHD continue to have symptoms into adulthood and many adults continue to derive benefits from taking stimulant medications to ameliorate their core symptoms of ADHD.[2]

Three aspects of ADHD have remained remarkably constant over the 35 to 40 years since it was first identified as MBD:

1

- **The diagnosis**: Although the name of the condition has been changed over time, the symptoms describing MBD are remarkably similar to that of ADHD-combined type, the current diagnosis.
- **The treatment**: Both stimulant medications and behavior modification were demonstrated to be efficacious treatments in rigorous controlled clinical trials undertaken in the early 1970s in children with ADHD, and those findings have been replicated in numerous additional studies over the subsequent years. In addition, medication has also been demonstrated to be efficacious in preschool-age children, adolescents, and adults.
- **The controversy**: Even as early as 1973, concern was raised that too many children were being treated with methylphenidate (MPH).[12] Challenges to the concept of ADHD as a valid condition and the concern about treatment with stimulant medications in particular have remained persistent (fueled by the media and certain religious groups) despite a large amount of scientific evidence to the contrary.

This book will provide the basic evidence that documents ADHD as a medical condition and its treatment. These facts will be used as the basis for recommending the current best practices for diagnosing and treating both children and adults.

REFERENCES

1. Jensen P, Cooper JR. *Attention Deficit Hyperactivity Disorder: State of Science Best Practices*. Kingstown, NJ: Civic Research Institute Inc; 2002.
2. Ingram S, Hechtman L, Morgenstern G. Outcome issues in ADHD: adolescent and adult long-term outcome. *Ment Retard Devel Disabil Res Rev.* 1999;5:243-250.
3. Hoffman H. *Der Struwewelpeter*. Leipzig, Germany: Imsel Verlag; 1848.
4. Still GF. Some abnormal physical conditions in children. The Goulstonian lectures. *Lancet.* 1902;1:1008-1012.
5. Hohman LB. Post-encephalitic behavior disorder in children. *Johns Hopkins Hosp Bull.* 1922;33:372-375.
6. Douglas VI, Peters KG. Toward a clearer definition of the attentional deficit of hyperactive children. In: Hale G, Lewis M, eds. *Attention and the Development of Cognitive Skills*. New York, NY: Plenum Press; 1978.
7. American Psychiatric Association. *Diagnostic and Statistical Manual for Mental Disorders.* 3rd ed. Washington, DC: American Psychiatric Association; 1980.
8. Wolraich ML, Lambert EW, Baumgaertel A, et al. Teachers' screening for attention deficit/hyperactivity disorder: comparing multinational samples on teacher ratings of ADHD. *J Abnorm Child Psychol*. 2003;31:445-455.
9. American Psychiatric Association. *Diagnostic and Statistical Manual of Mental Disorders.* 3rd ed rev. Washington, DC: American Psychiatric Association; 1987.
10. American Psychiatric Association. *Diagnostic and Statistical Manual of Mental Disorders.* 4th ed. Washington, DC: American Psychiatric Association; 1994.
11. Wolraich ML, Hannah JN, Pinnock TY, Baumgaertel A, Brown J. Comparison of diagnostic criteria for attention-deficit hyperactivity disorder in a county-wide sample. *J Am Acad Child Adolesc Psychiatry*. 1996;35:319-324.
12. Maynard R. Omaha pupils given "behavior" drugs. *The Washington Post.* June 29, 1970.

2

Etiology, Prevalence, and Long-Term Outcomes

2

Etiology

ADHD is a heterogeneous disorder in that several etiologic pathways can manifest in a similar behavioral presentation. Although brain damage due to prematurity or birth trauma was initially thought to be the most common cause of ADHD (see Chapter 1, *Introduction and History*), the most common cause by far is genetic transmission. This is most clearly demonstrated in twin studies that have found heritability rates as high as 0.75 (ie, 75% of the variance in phenotype can be attributed to genetic factors).[1] Family studies have also shown that adoptive relatives of children with ADHD are less likely to have the disorder than biologic relatives,[2] biologic siblings are at a two- to three-times greater risk,[3] and first-degree relatives are at greater risk compared with controls.[4] Most recently, specific gene associations have been identified in a portion of individuals with ADHD. These include the dopamine transporter gene (DAT1),[5] the D4 receptor gene (DRD4),[6] and the human thyroid receptor gene.[7]

While the genetic component is the most common etiology, insults to the brain can also result in the behaviors that are characteristic of ADHD. There is a higher incidence of ADHD, as well as learning disabilities, in children who are born prematurely.[8] Traumatic injuries to the brain can also result in similar behavioral patterns.[8] Exposures in utero, particularly to alcohol, can cause ADHD symptomatology that in its severe form, is manifested as fetal alcohol syndrome. Infections, such as meningitis in young children, or exposures to lead or nicotine can also result in similar behavioral symptoms.[8]

Progress has also been made in identifying some of the preliminary central nervous system (CNS) mechanisms. Studies of brain anatomy have demonstrated that on average, individuals with ADHD have smaller prefrontal cortex, basal ganglia, and cerebellar vermix than do matched controls.[9] Functional studies, such as positron emission tomography, single-photon emission computed tomography (SPECT), and functional magnetic resonance imaging (fMRI), have shown striatal hypoperfusion in populations with ADHD compared with controls.[9] The affected brain areas are clearly related to the dopamine and norepinephrine systems. A recent longitudinal imaging study found that the differences in cortical maturation between individuals with ADHD and a comparison group disappeared by the age of 25 years.[10] It is important to note that differences in brain volumes between those with ADHD and matched controls were not caused by exposure to stimulant medications.[8,9] It is also important to note that while research has progressed significantly in helping to identify possible underlying mechanisms in individuals with ADHD, the sophisticated assessment techniques now available do not help facilitate the clinical diagnosis. There is such wide variation in individuals with and without ADHD, both in the size and activity of the brain (with a good deal of overlap between the two groups), that the assessments cannot adequately diagnose individuals with ADHD.

In children, the diagnosis of ADHD remains dependent on the reports of those who most closely observe the children—parents and teachers. In adults, self reports and those of spouses, significant-other relationships, and other family members can be helpful. As with other mental disorders, the diagnosis is made based on the presence of specific behaviors or symptoms that occur for a defined minimal amount of time and cause impairment. As such, it is the same process that is used for other mental disorders, such as depression or schizophrenia, for which a clinical interview is diagnostic.

Prevalence

Determining the true prevalence rate of ADHD has been a challenging task. It is also a main source of controversy in the popular press, in which it is frequently asserted that too many individuals are diagnosed with ADHD and treated with stimulant medication. Four characteristics of the disorder contribute to the difficulties in determining the true prevalence:

- The diagnosis is dependent on the presence of specific behaviors that are observed and reported, in the case of children, by the child's caregivers or in adults, self reported, or reported by individuals close to the patients. Since there are no specific biologic markers (lab tests or image studies), the diagnosis must rely on the subjective judgment of these reporters. The judgments are also subjective because there are no clear normative criteria about what frequency of any given behavior is normal for any given age. Other assessments, such as determining intelligence, have clear normative guidelines for what tasks can be accomplished at any given age, requiring less subjective judgment. These judgments are likely to be affected by the circumstances under which the individual is observed and the cultural norms of both the patient and the reporters, such as parents, teachers, social workers, psychologists, and physicians.
- The second feature is that there is no clear demarcation between appropriate and inappropriate behaviors. For example, symptoms of hallucinations or delusions are clear manifestations of psychotic disorders that are not generally found in individuals who do not have some disorder. However, the behaviors in ADHD occur in a more normative distribution, so some defined cutoff point has to be set in order to establish diagnostic criteria. This phenomenon creates challenges for primary care clinicians, who are the physicians most likely to see those cases that are of milder severity and may be on the borderline for diagnosis.
- The third feature is that determining the presence of the behaviors and their impact, particularly in children, is dependent on reports from parents and teachers where there frequently is disagreement between the two sources. The disagreement does not necessarily reflect inaccurate reporting on the part of either teachers or parents.[11] Teachers frequently see children in situations where they need to focus and pay attention because of the nature of

the tasks. At home, there is less pressure on children to concentrate, and there is usually a much higher adult-to-child ratio than occurs at school. Teachers also have the advantage of concurrently observing a much greater number of same-age peers under similar circumstances, which they can use as a comparison group.

- The changes in criteria over time have further complicated the process of determining the true prevalence of ADHD. The most recent change from only one subtype in *DSM-IIIR* to three subtypes in *DSM-IV* has been associated with increases in the prevalence rates (**Figure 2.1**).[12] The requirement of some hyperactivity or impulsivity as a diagnostic criterion when there was only one subtype resulted in a number of individuals not considered as having ADHD despite their difficulties with inattention and organizational skills. The older criteria likely excluded more females, who more frequently do not manifest hyperactive behavior.

Besides the challenges in making accurate diagnoses, studies of prevalence rates are dependent on the sample

FIGURE 2.1 — Percentage of Patients Meeting ADHD Core Symptom Requirements in Epidemiologic Studies (1994)

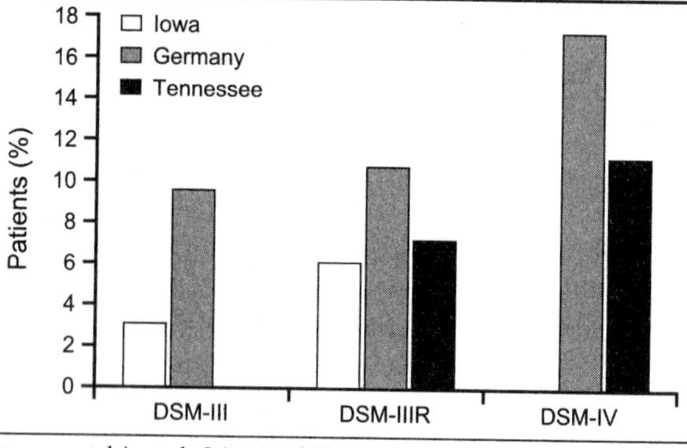

Baumgaertel A, et al. *J Am Acad Child Adolesc Psychiatry*. 1995;34:629-638.

studied. The rates are different when one examines a mental health clinic–referred sample in comparison to a primary care sample or a community/school sample. Given these challenges, it is not surprising that there are varying rates. The prevalence has ranged from 4% to 12% (median 5.8%).[13] Rates are higher in community samples (10.3%) compared with school samples (6.9%), higher in males (9.2%) than females (3.0%), and higher with the changes in diagnostic criteria (*DSM-III>IIIR>IV*). There is a preponderance of males in the range of 3 to 4 to 1.[14] The gender differences are less for the inattentive type where there is a 2 to 1 ratio.[15]

A recent Centers for Disease Control (CDC) study utilized district-wide school-based screenings of >11,000 elementary students (kindergarten through fifth grade) in four districts to develop strata of probable cases (high-screen) and probable controls (low-screen) that were then more extensively evaluated with structured psychiatric interviews to determine which children met a rigorous study-based case definition for ADHD, including symptom and impairment criteria from teacher screening data. Weighted percentages meeting the case definition of ADHD were: 10.1% of White and 12.1% of African American students.[16] In adults who have been diagnosed with ADHD as children, 50% to 70% continue to show impairment.[17] Population studies in adults demonstrate a prevalence rate of 4.4%.[18]

Further complicating the determination of prevalence is that at any given time, there are a number of individuals with ADHD on treatment with stimulant medications. It is frequently not possible to determine retrospectively how many of these individuals were accurately diagnosed and no longer had symptoms because of effective treatment or how many were inappropriately diagnosed and were being needlessly treated with medication. In the CDC study cited here, an additional 5.4% of the White and 4.1% of the African American students were in those categories. In addition, 17.2% of those White students who were being treated with medication and 49.9% of those African American students still demonstrated sufficient symptoms to meet diagnostic criteria despite treatment. The results suggest that there are still many children with ADHD who continue to go undiagnosed and treated; in addition, a significant number of those treated are not sufficiently treated to reduce their symptoms to within the normal range. Furthermore, African American children are less likely to be diagnosed and treated, and their treatment is more likely to inadequately reduce their symptoms.[16]

Long-Term Outcomes

It is clear that ADHD is a condition with significant consequences for those affected. Individuals with ADHD are at considerable risk for having long-term problems due to their condition, particularly if they do not receive treatment. While it was once believed that the condition resolved by puberty, it is now clear that the majority of individuals with ADHD will continue to manifest symptoms and have significant impairments as adults.[19] The initial observations probably related to the fact that many of the individuals with ADHD who manifested hyperactive behaviors as children no longer manifested those behaviors as adults. It is now recognized, however, that many adolescents and adults continue to report sensations of restlessness and difficulty in sitting through meetings. The manifestations of inattention and disorganization typically persist into adulthood, and some data suggest that ADHD is more functionally impairing than most other outpatient psychiatric conditions.[19]

Long-term follow-up studies of individuals with ADHD have demonstrated poorer outcomes in a number of domains. As occurs in childhood, academic performance continues to be a prominent impairment in adults.[20] They also have more difficulties with peer and marital relations,[20] greater rates of motor vehicular accidents and violations,[21] greater rates of substance abuse,[22] and more legal difficulties. Sixty-nine percent of the children with ADHD will continue to have symptoms in adulthood.[23]

ADHD is a highly prevalent condition in both children and adults and is caused primarily by genetic factors, although insults to the brain during gestation or after birth can be causes or contributing factors. The symptoms frequently continue into adulthood and frequently cause significant disabilities if untreated.

REFERENCES

1. Waldman I, Rhee SH. Behavioural and molecular genetic studies. In: Sandberg S, ed. *Hyperactivity and Attention Disorders in Childhood.* 2nd ed. Cambridge, UK: Cambridge University Press; 2002:290-335.
2. Alberts-Corush J, Firestone P, Goodman JT. Attention and impulsivity characteristics of the biological and adoptive parents of hyperactive and normal control children. *Am J Orthopsychiatry.* 1986;56:413-423.
3. Biederman J, Faraone SV, Keenan K, Knee D, Tsuang MT. Family-genetic and psychosocial risk factors in DSM-III attention deficit disorder. *J Am Acad Child Adolesc Psychiatry.* 1990;29: 526-533.
4. Cantwell DP. Psychiatric illness in the families of hyperactive children. *Arch Gen Psychiatry.* 1972;27:414-417.
5. Waldman ID, Rowe DC, Abramowitz A, et al. Association and linkage of the dopamine transporter gene and attention-deficit hyperactivity disorder in children: heterogeneity owing to diagnostic subtype and severity. *Am J Hum Genet.* 1998;63:1767-1776.
6. Swanson JM, Sunohara GA, Kennedy JL, et al. Association of the dopamine receptor D4 (DRD4) gene with a refined phenotype of attention deficit hyperactivity disorder (ADHD): a family-based approach. *Mol Psychiatry.* 1998;3:38-41.
7. Hauser P, Zametkin AJ, Martinez P, et al. Attention deficit-hyperactivity disorder in people with generalized resistance to thyroid hormone. *N Engl J Med.* 1993;328:997-1001.
8. Swanson J, Castellanos FX. Biological bases of ADHD: neuroanatomy, genetics, and pathophysiology. In: Jensen PS, Cooper JR, eds. *Attention Deficit Hyperactivity Disorder: State of the Science—Best Practices.* Kingston, NJ: Civic Research Institute; 2002:7-1-7-20.
9. Kelly AM, Margulies DS, Castellanos FX. Recent advances in structural and functional brain imaging studies of attention-deficit/hyperactivity disorder. *Curr Psychiatry Rep.* 2007;9:401-407.
10. Shaw P, Eckstrand K, Sharp W, et al. Attention-deficit/hyperactivity disorder is characterized by a delay in cortical maturation. *Proc Natl Acad Sci USA.* 2007;104:19649-19654.
11. Wolraich ML, Lambert EW, Bickman L, Simmons T, Doffing MA, Worley KA. Assessing the impact of parent and teacher agreement on diagnosing attention-deficit hyperactivity disorder. *J Dev Behav Pediatr.* 2004;25:41-47.

12. Baumgaertel A, Wolraich ML, Dietrich M. Comparison of diagnostic criteria for attention deficit disorders in a German elementary school sample. *J Am Acad Child Adolesc Psychiatry.* 1995;34:629-638.

13. Brown RT, Freeman WS, Perrin JM, et al. Prevalence and assessment of attention-deficit/hyperactivity disorder in primary care settings. *Pediatrics.* 2001;107:E43.

14. Gaub M, Carlson CL. Gender differences in ADHD: a meta-analysis and critical review. *J Am Acad Child Adolesc Psychiatry.* 1997;36:1036-1045.

15. Wolraich ML, Hannah JN, Pinnock TY, Baumgaertel A, Brown J. Comparison of diagnostic criteria for attention-deficit hyperactivity disorder in a county-wide sample. *J Am Acad Child Adolesc Psychiatry.* 1996;35:319-324.

16. Wolraich M, MeKeown RE, Visser S, PLAY Collaborative. Prevalence of ADHD in a Community Sample. Annual Pediatric Academic Societies Meeting. Honolulu, HI; May 2-6, 2008.

17. Faraone SV, Biederman J, Mick E. The age-dependent decline of attention deficit hyperactivity disorder: a meta-analysis of follow-up studies. *Psychol Med.* 2006;36:159-165.

18. Kessler R. Prevalence of Adult ADHD in the United States: Results from the National Comorbidity Study Replication (NCS-R). Paper presented at: 157th American Psychiatric Association Annual Meeting; New York, NY; May 1-6, 2004.

19. Barkley RA, Murphy KR, Fischer M. *ADHD in Adults: What the Science Says*. New York, NY: Guilford Press; 2007.

20. Barkley RA, Fischer M, Smallish L, Fletcher K. Young adult outcome of hyperactive children: adaptive functioning in major life activities. *J Am Acad Child Adolesc Psychiatry*. 2006;45:192-202.

21. Barkley RA, Murphy KR, Dupaul GI, Bush T. Driving in young adults with attention deficit hyperactivity disorder: knowledge, performance, adverse outcomes, and the role of executive functioning. *J Int Neuropsychol Soc*. 2002;8:655-672.

22. Compton WM, Thomas YF, Stinson FS, Grant BF. Prevalence, correlates, disability, and comorbidity of DSM-IV drug abuse and dependence in the United States: results from the national epidemiologic survey on alcohol and related conditions. *Arch Gen Psychiatry*. 2007;64:566-576.

23. Biederman J, Petty CR, Fried R, et al. Stability of executive function deficits into young adult years: a prospective longitudinal follow-up study of grown up males with ADHD. *Acta Psychiatr Scand.* 2007;116:129-136.

3 Diagnosis of ADHD

Specific Criteria

The diagnosis of ADHD has been somewhat challenging because there are no pathognomonic tests available to establish a definitive diagnosis. It is based on the report of the presence of specific behaviors that impair an individual's functioning. Therefore, to make the diagnosis of ADHD, the clinician needs to determine the presence of behaviors as outlined by the most recent changes in criteria in the *Diagnostic and Statistical Manual of Mental Disorders, 4th Edition, Text Revision* (*DSM-IV-TR*).[1] These criteria now include two dimensions: inattention and hyperactivity/impulsivity. From these two dimensions, three subtypes have been derived. The behaviors specific to each dimension are characterized in **Table 3.1**. The clinician needs to determine how many of the core symptoms are occurring more often than what would be expected for the patient's developmental level, and the extent that these symptoms cause dysfunction in more than one setting, particularly at home and in school, as well as at work for adolescents and adults.

To be considered as having the necessary symptoms in each dimension, an individual must display at least six of nine of the dimension's behaviors "inappropriately often for the developmental level of the individual."

Sources of Information

The diagnosis of ADHD remains dependent on obtaining information about a patient's behavior from those who most frequently observe the behavior. For children, the sources need to include their parents and teachers, at a minimum. Teachers observe children for up to 6 hours a day in situations that require the children to pay attention and control their activity level and impulsivity, and they are able to observe them among a group of same-age peers. In fact, the American Academy of

TABLE 3.1 — Core Symptoms of ADHD

Inattention Dimension

- Careless mistakes
- Difficulty sustaining attention
- Seems not to listen
- Fails to finish tasks
- Difficulty organizing
- Avoids tasks requiring sustained attention
- Loses things
- Easily distracted
- Forgetful

Hyperactivity-Impulsivity Dimension

- Hyperactivity:
  - Fidgeting
  - Unable to stay seated
  - Moving excessively (restless)
  - Difficulty engaging in leisure activities quietly
  - "On the go"
  - Talking excessively
- Impulsivity:
  - Blurting answers before questions completed
  - Difficulty awaiting turn
  - Interrupting/intruding upon others

Pediatrics (AAP) guidelines recommend that obtaining information from teachers, as well as parents, is essential in making the diagnosis.[2] Where possible, it is also helpful to obtain information from other observers, such as coaches, scout leaders, and grandparents. Direct observations of a child's behavior in the classroom can provide some of the most objective information if it is available, but it is labor intensive and therefore can only capture a limited amount of observed time. A diagnostic algorithm for ADHD in children and adolescents is presented in **Figure 3.1**.

For adolescents and adults, it is more difficult to obtain the information from sources other than the patient. Unfortunately, in adolescents as in younger children, they may be unreliable reporters of their own behavior.[3] However, parents frequently have fewer opportunities to observe their children, and by middle school and high school, students frequently have multiple teachers who only observe them for limited times each

FIGURE 3.1 — ADHD Diagnostic Algorithm for Children and Adolescents

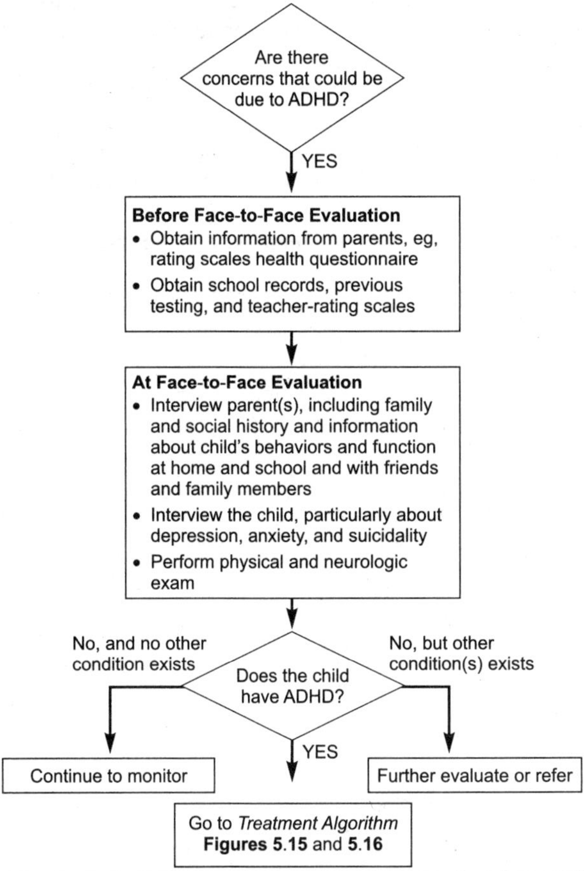

day. When possible, it is still best to have both teacher and parent input. It is also important to determine how well the adolescent is able to monitor their own behavior.

The process of assessing adults is usually based solely on the report of the patient. However, the clinician should keep in mind that the evidence indicates that adults,[4] just as with children[5] and adolescents,[3] may not be accurate reporters. When possible, it is helpful to get additional information from other family members or significant others. **Figure 3.2** shows a diagnostic algorithm for ADHD in adults.

In the assessment of children, there frequently is disagreement between parents and teachers.[6] To a great degree, the disagreement relates to the different situations in which teachers and parents observe the child. When there is significant disagreement, it is helpful to try and determine who is providing the most accurate perceptions. Biases can be present with the parent, the

FIGURE 3.2 — ADHD Diagnostic Algorithm for Adults

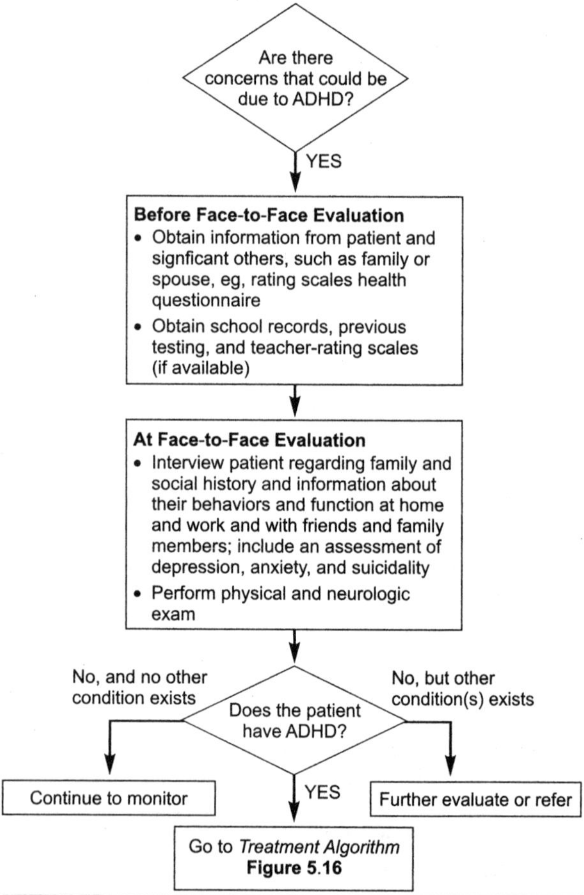

teacher, or both. Some suggestions on how to clarify the differences are presented in **Table 3.2**.

Other Criteria

In addition to the core symptoms, patients with the diagnosis must meet the following other criteria presented in **Table 3.3**.

Depending on which core symptoms are present, ADHD contains three subtypes:

- *Predominantly inattentive type*, individuals who meet the criteria on the inattentive dimension (six or more of nine inattentive core symptoms);

TABLE 3.2 — Evaluating Reporter Disagreement of ADHD Symptoms in Children

- Review the behaviors at least with the parent to ensure that they are accurately observing the specific behaviors.
- Obtain information from additional sources, including previous teachers, current ancillary teachers, aides, coaches, scout or organizational leaders, religious teachers, the other parent or step-parent, and other relatives.
- Getting a report of the child's behavior during psychoeducational counseling can also be illuminating.
- Determine if the parents or the teachers are strongly opinionated either for or against medication.
- Determine if the differences are due to differences in how reporters completed the scales, such as their interpretation of the frequencies of reported behaviors.
- Determine cultural differences.

TABLE 3.3 — Other Criteria Required for the Diagnosis of ADHD

- Some hyperactive-impulsive or inattentive symptoms that caused impairment present before 7 years of age
- Symptoms have persisted for at least 6 months
- Some impairment from the symptoms is present in two or more settings (eg, home, school, or work).
- Evidence for significant clinical impairment in social, academic, or occupational functioning due to the behavior.

- *Predominantly hyperactive-impulsive type*, individuals who meet the criteria on the hyperactivity-impulsivity dimension (six or more of nine hyperactive/impulsive core symptoms);
- *Combined type*, individuals who meet the criteria (six of nine) on both dimensions.

The requirement of the age of 7 years is included to reflect a biologic basis for the condition starting in childhood. The age is not empirically derived, and there is some debate that some children with the inattentive subtype may not present until an older age, when they have a greater need to be able to concentrate. The requirement of at least 6 months' duration reflects the chronic nature of the condition. The most important aspect of the diagnosis is the concept that the core symptoms impair the patient's ability to function. There are individuals who have many of the core symptoms, but because of their strengths (eg, above-average intelligence), they are able to compensate well enough to prevent the symptoms from causing significant dysfunction.

Based on *DSM-IV*, a diagnosis of ADHD should not be made in those with a diagnosis of pervasive developmental disorders (autism) or childhood schizophrenia. However, children with autism may display a number of core symptoms of ADHD, and although it is less likely that there will be a beneficial response, some will improve on medications used to treat ADHD. Other conditions, such as mood and anxiety disorders and learning disabilities, may cause ADHD symptoms, but these are also common comorbid conditions.

Challenges in Establishing the Diagnosis

The current diagnostic criteria for ADHD are less than perfect even if they are the state-of-the-art criteria. First, the *DSM* system does not include a developmental perspective. The diagnostic criteria were derived primarily from research in children 6 to 13 years of age. In adolescents and adults, the clinician frequently is trying to base a diagnosis on retrospective recall of the patient to determine if the diagnosis occurred in childhood. The 18 core symptoms are derived from field trials in children ranging from 4 to 17 years of age and some of the behaviors are not appropriately worded for adults, such as "runs or climbs excessively."[7] Some have also argued that the criteria of six core symptoms in one of the dimensions is overly restrictive for adults.[8] The number of ADHD symptoms declines in the general population with increasing age, and adults with four to five ADHD symptoms in one category are likely to be significantly different from age-normed peers.[9]

3

The behaviors are also contextually dependent. The greater the adult-child ratio for children, the stronger the interest the individual has, or the greater the structure in the environment, the easier it is for an individual to control his/her behaviors. There are also no specific guidelines for an observer, such as a parent or teacher, to precisely decide that a behavior is occurring inappropriately often. Therefore, the reporting of the symptoms is to some extent subjective, and the finding mentioned earlier about discrepancies between parent and teacher reports are not surprising. Generally, teacher reports have correlated well with direct observations of the children in the classroom.[10] The teachers' reports will be more accurate in elementary school where a teacher is likely to have a child for a good portion of the day. It is more difficult in middle and high school where teachers may only have a student for 45 minutes each day. It is helpful to gather as much information as possible from multiple sources—at least from both the parents and teachers.

An additional challenge is that the behaviors are not an all-or-none phenomenon. Some of the behaviors may be normally expected, depending on the age of the child and the circumstance. Children with difficult temperaments may have some difficulties that create problems, but their symptoms, and more important, their degree of dysfunction, are not severe enough to warrant a diagnosis of ADHD. These have been referred to as "subsyndromal" and are defined in the *DSM for Primary Care Child and Adolescent Version*[11] as inattentive and hyperactive/impulsive problems. While treatment with medication is not appropriate for this group of children, behavioral interventions are appropriate. Close monitoring is important because some of these children will become disordered as the environmental demands increase with age.

Many of the behaviors will decrease with age, so in adolescents and adults, it is less common to see the hyperactive and impulse symptoms. However, engaging in quiet leisure activities, and interrupting other people can persist.[8] The symptoms of inattention and difficulties with executive function while also diminishing are likely to continue into adulthood, although some of the patients are successful at accommodating for these deficits as they mature. Problems that frequently persist are paying close attention to details, sustaining attention with tasks, and following through on instructions.[8]

It is important to obtain enough information to make a diagnosis based on *DSM-IV* criteria. Using rating scales that base their behavioral symptoms on *DSM-IV* can help to shorten the time required to obtain the information (**Table 3.4**). This fact is particularly true in obtaining information from teachers, where direct contact may be difficult. There are several scales available, including the Vanderbilt Parent and Teacher ADHD Rating Scale,[12] the SNAP-IV,[13] the DuPaul Parent and Teacher Rating Scales,[14] and the Revised Conners Teacher and Parent Rating Scales. All of the listed scales, with the exception of the Revised Conners Teacher and Parent Rating Scale and the DuPaul Parent Rating Scale, are in the public domain. Website information is provided in **Table 3.4**,

TABLE 3.4 — *DSM-IV*–Based ADHD Rating Scales for Children and Adolescents

- Vanderbilt
  - http://devbehavpeds.ouhsc.edu/rokplay.asp
- SNAP-IV
  - www.adhd.net
- DuPaul ADHD Rating Scale IV
  - http://www.guilfordpress.co.uk/adhd.asp
- Conners Rating Scales, Revised
  - http://portal.wpspublish.com/portal/page?_pageid=53,112710&_dad=portal&_schema=PORTAL

Accessed March 30, 2009.

and the Vanderbilt Scales with scoring instructions are provided in an appendix at the end of this book.

Other tests have not been found to be useful in making the diagnosis. It is important to screen children with ADHD for lead, as would be done for other children if they are living in an at-risk area. Computerized electroencephalogram (EEG) assessments are utilized for research purposes but have not been found to contribute to making a diagnosis.[15] Similarly, MRI and SPECT scans have not been shown to be diagnostic of ADHD in individual patients.[15]

3

Many children with ADHD will also have poor coordination in fine and/or gross motor skills. These findings used to be called "soft neurologic signs" because part of the manifestation was the retention of signs (such as overflow activity) beyond the expected age at which they should disappear. Deficits in coordination have been referred to as developmental coordination disorder or motor dysfunction. They are important to identify because they can impair social functions, such as the child's performance in sporting activities, and they can impair academic performance in writing (referred to by the school system as written expression).

An assessment of functioning is a required component in establishing the diagnosis. The second section of the Vanderbilt Parent and Teacher ADHD rating scales provides information about functioning. The SNAP is usually administered with the Swanson, Kotin, Atkins, M-Flynn, and Pelham (SKAMP) rating scale that assesses function, and the SKAMP is available from the same source as the SNAP. In addition, both the parent and child should be asked about how well the child is doing in the domains of peer and family relations and academic, community (organized activities), and leisure functioning.

The rating scales used for children are generally acceptable for use in adolescents. However, the Conners Adolescent ADHD scale is more specific for this population. In adults, the most useful scales are versions of the *DSM-IV* criteria, such as the Barkley version, the Conners Adult ADHD Rating Scale (CAARS),[16] and the Adult Self-Rating Scale (ASRS) produced by the World

Health Organization (**Table 3.5**).[17] Tom Brown, PhD, has published a scale for assessment of the inattentive symptoms in adults, the Brown Adults Attention Disorder Scale (BAADS).[18]

A common practice is to have the adult and any collateral raters complete one of these rating scales twice: once to assess current symptoms and the second time in retrospect to assess for symptoms as a child or adolescent. Paul Wender has developed a scale to help evaluate adults for the assessment of the childhood symptoms retrospectively.[19]

There are a number of conditions that can cause symptoms that may mimic those of ADHD. These physical and psychological conditions may be the causes of the ADHD symptoms and are therefore important to diagnose if present. However, it is crucial to recognize that these conditions can also occur as comorbid conditions in those who also have ADHD. At times, this differentiation can be challenging.

A careful history, physical exam, and lab testing as necessary are helpful to rule out physical disorders such as lead toxicity, medication toxicities, sleep disorders (eg, obstructive sleep apnea), seizure disorders, closed head injuries, CNS disorders (eg, Wilson's disease, multiple sclerosis, sickle cell anemia), learning disorders, cognitive impairments (eg, fragile X syndrome, cerebral palsy, Klinefelter's syndrome), and pervasive developmental disorders, such as autism. In addition, anxiety, depression, and bipolar disorders can mimic symptoms of ADHD. If

TABLE 3.5 — *DSM-IV*–Based Rating Scales for Adults

- Brown Adult ADD Scale
  - http://pearsonassessment.com (type "Brown ADD Scale" in search box)
- Conners Adult ADD Scale
  - https://www.mhs.com/ecom/(3czddrmy4fm1yjn05qj0air3)/product.aspx?RptGrpID=CAA
- Conners Adolescent ADD Scale
  - https://www.mhs.com/ecom/(3czddrmy4fm1yjn05qj0air3)/product.aspx?RptGrpID=C3A

Accessed March 30, 2009.

the symptoms of ADHD predate the symptoms of anxiety or depression, it is likely that the individual can be diagnosed with both conditions. However, if the symptoms of ADHD began at the same time as did those of the psychologic disorder, it is more likely that the symptoms of ADHD are caused by anxiety or depression.

Diagnosis of Comorbid Conditions

Because co-occurring conditions, both behavioral and physical, are common in patients with ADHD, it is important that clinicians not only determine that a patient has ADHD and does not have another condition that better explains the current symptoms; but they also need to determine if other conditions are present. Comorbidity is the term that the *DSM-IV* uses to refer to disorders that are present at the same time as the ADHD and are not the cause of the ADHD symptoms. The majority of individuals with ADHD will have at least one comorbid condition.

The comorbid conditions can be categorized into four groups:

- Learning and language disorders
- Externalizing conditions
- Internalizing conditions
- Motoric and physical disorders.

■ Learning and Language Disorders

Learning disorders are specific cognitive deficits that interfere with some aspects of learning or academic performance such that the individual is not able to achieve up to their overall cognitive ability. The deficits can be in any academic activity (eg, reading, written expression, or mathematics), although the most common disability is in reading. Individuals with learning disabilities in reading (dyslexia) most frequently have a weakness in their ability to discriminate the sounds in words, referred to as phonologic awareness. A language deficit is also frequently associated with the disability. Learning disorders can be suspected even before children start school if the children appear delayed in learning their letters or colors. The previous idea that letter reversal was the major characteristic of a learning disability is not correct as some mild continuation of letter reversal or substitute letters in children who do not have learning disabilities is seen. The language disorders frequently are related to the practical use of language, referred to as pragmatics, and may not be detected with traditional speech and language evaluations

If a learning or language disorder is suspected, the patient should receive a psychoeducational battery of tests to characterize their cognitive and academic skills. It should include, at a minimum, a standardized individual general test of intelligence, such as the Wechsler Intelligence Scale for Children, 4th Edition (WISC-IV), and an individualized standard achievement test, such as the Woodcock Johnson III Test of Achievement, Revised. It is important to get a speech and language evaluation as well if a language disorder is considered. The Wechsler Adult Intelligence Scale (WAIS) is usually only used for adults. The assessment can be obtained through the school system at no charge to the family or by referral to a learning clinic, psychologist, or school performance clinic. An informal screen can be used initially by determining a child's grades and annual group achievement tests, and then checking with the parents and teachers to determine if they think the child is performing satisfactorily and up to his/her potential. It is helpful to know the school system's procedures regarding assessing children. Given the demands that some schools face with limited funding, it may take some prodding by the parents to ensure that their child is evaluated in a timely fashion. Parents or caregivers may need to make the requests for service in writing and becoming knowledgeable about the rules and regulations present in the school district.

Those who are no longer in school will need to be assessed by a psychologist if this testing is considered warranted. Children or adolescents who are underperforming in school should have psychoeducational testing. The decision to test adults is typically made on a case-by-case basis.

Impaired cognitive abilities that in the past were referred to as mental retardation are not a contraindication for diagnosing or treating a child with ADHD.[20] Stimulant medications can be beneficial for children with intellectual disabilities and ADHD although they are not as efficacious in those individuals with more severe limitations.[21]

■ Other Behavioral Disorders

Broad-based rating scales (such as the Conners Parent and Teacher Rating Scales, the Child Behavior Checklist [CBCL] for parents and teachers and Youth Form), Behavioral Assessment System for Children, 2nd Edition (BASC-2), and specific scales (eg Multidimensional Anxiety Scale for Children and the Children's Depression Inventory) can be helpful in identifying possible comorbid conditions.

3

Externalizing Conditions

The next most common group of behavioral comorbid conditions are the externalizing conditions. In addition to ADHD, the other externalizing conditions are oppositional defiant disorder (ODD) and conduct disorder (CD). ODD is a milder manifestation of CD and is frequently the first presentation seen in children who subsequently develop CD. Its symptoms are presented in **Table 3.6**. They reflect poor control of anger and defiance. A child must have at least four of the eight symptoms, which must be present for at least 6 months, and they must cause clinically significant impairment. The symptoms may diminish as the child's ADHD is treated with stimulant medication. However, parents and teachers may require some training in behavior management to adequately deal with the child.

CD is essentially a more severe manifestation of antisocial behaviors and is characterized by behaviors that violate the rights of others and the norms of society. The specific behaviors are presented in **Table 3.7**. Three of these behaviors occurring in the past year with at least one in the past 6 months causing significant impairment are required to make the diagnosis.

The disturbances in behavior must cause clinically significant impairment in social, academic, or occupational functioning. Conduct disorder is not diagnosed if the individual is >18 years of age and meets the criteria for antisocial personality disorder. Children or adoles-

TABLE 3.6 — *DSM-IV* Criteria for Oppositional Defiant Disorder

A pattern of negativistic, hostile, and defiant behavior lasting at least 6 months and having at least four of the following symptoms present at a frequency that is greater than typically observed in individuals of similar age and development level:

- Loses temper
- Argues with adult
- Actively defies or refuses to comply with requests or rules of adults
- Deliberately annoys people
- Blames others for his/her mistakes or behavior
- Touchy or easily annoyed by others
- Angry or resentful
- Spiteful or vindictive

cents with CD have more significant problems with comorbidity with both ADHD and depression. They are also at greater risk for substance abuse, and 25% to 40% eventually develop antisocial personality disorder as an adult. Many will require intense coordinated services, such as multisystem therapy.

Internalizing Conditions

Mood Disorders

The mood disorders are primarily characterized by major depressive episodes, manic episodes, and anxiety disorders. Major depressive episodes are characterized by the symptoms described in **Table 3.8**. One or more major depressive episodes will occur in a major depressive disorder. However, if the symptoms are more chronic (ie, lasting at least 2 years) and there are symptoms (two or more), but no major depressive episodes, the condition is referred to as a dysthymic disorder.

If the major depressive episodes are present between manic episodes (**Table 3.9**), a patient has a bipolar disorder. Sometimes an individual may have manic episodes without depression initially and may appear to have ADHD. A family history of bipolar disorder places an individual at higher risk, so the clinician should have a greater sensitivity to the possibility of bipolar disorder if the patient has a positive family history. One or more

TABLE 3.7 — *DSM-IV* Criteria for Conduct Disorder

A repetitive and persistent pattern of behavior in which the basic rights of others or age-appropriate societal norms or rules are violated. This disorder is manifested by the presence of three or more of the following criteria occurring in the past 12 months with at least one criterion present in the past 6 months:

- Aggression to people and animals
  - Bullies, threatens, or intimidates others
  - Initiates physical fights
  - Has used a weapon that can cause serious physical harm to others
  - Has been physically cruel to people
  - Has been physically cruel to animals
  - Has stolen while confronting a victim
  - Has forced someone into sexual activity
- Destruction of property
  - Has deliberately engaged in fire-setting with intent to cause serious damage
  - Has deliberately destroyed others' property (other than by fire-setting)
- Deceitfulness or theft
  - Has broken into someone else's house, building, or car
  - Lies to obtain goods or favors or to avoid obligations (ie, "cons" others)
  - Has stolen items of value without confronting a victim (eg, shoplifting)
- Serious violations of rules
  - Stays out at night despite parental prohibitions, beginning before age 13
  - Has run away from home overnight at least twice (or once without returning for a lengthy period)
  - Often truant from school, beginning before age 13

major depressive episodes will occur in a major depressive disorder. However, if the symptoms are more chronic (ie, lasting at least 2 years) and there are symptoms (two or more), but no major depressive episodes, the condition is referred to as a dysthymic disorder.

The symptoms of bipolar depression are less clear in children than they are in adolescents and adults. There remain disagreements about the extent to which bipolar disorder occurs in school-age children. However, it is important to consider in children with a strong family

TABLE 3.8 — *DSM-IV* Criteria for Major Depressive Episode

Five (or more) of the following symptoms have been present during the same 2-week period and represent a change from previous functioning; at least one of the symptoms is either depressed mood or loss of interest or pleasure:

- Depressed mood most of the day, nearly every day (in children and adolescents, can be irritable mood)
- Markedly diminished interest or pleasure in all, or almost all, activities most of the day, every day
- Significant weight loss when not dieting or weight gain or increase in appetite. (Note: In children, consider failure to make expected weight gains.)
- Insomnia or hypersomnia nearly every day
- Psychomotor agitation or retardation nearly every day
- Fatigue or loss of energy nearly every day
- Feelings of worthlessness or excessive or inappropriate guilt
- Diminished ability to think or concentrate, or indecisiveness, nearly every day
- Recurrent thoughts of death (not just fear of dying)

TABLE 3.9 — *DSM-IV* Criteria for Manic Episode

During the period of mood disturbance, three (or more) of the following symptoms have persisted (four if the mood is only irritable) and have been present to a significant degree:

- Inflated self-esteem or grandiosity
- Decreased need for sleep (eg, feels rested after only 3 hours of sleep)
- More talkative than usual or pressure to keep talking
- Flight of ideas
- Racing of thoughts
- Distractibility (ie, attention too easily drawn to unimportant or irrelevant external stimuli)
- Increase in goal-directed activity (either socially, at work or school, or sexually)
- Psychomotor agitation
- Excessive involvement in pleasurable activities

history and in those who are unresponsive to ADHD treatments and include a good deal of anger, irritability, and oppositional behavior.

Anxiety Disorders

Phobias are marked, persistent, and excessive or unreasonable fears of specific types of situations (eg, animal, natural environment, the sight of blood or receiving injections) or of social situations (social phobias). Exposure to the phobic stimulus causes an immediate anxiety response even though the individual realizes that the response is excessive or unreasonable.

3

Panic attacks are discrete periods of intense fear or discomfort of sudden onset. They reach a peak within 10 minutes and are characterized by autonomic responses including palpitations, tachycardia, sweating, cold or hot flushes, and trembling. The individual may experience shortness of breath, chest pain, abdominal distress, dizziness, and parethesias. They fear losing control or dying or feel "unreal."

Posttraumatic Stress Disorder (PTSD)

The diagnosis of PTSD requires the patient to have experienced or witnessed an event that involves actual or threatened serious injury or death. The event needs to be persistently reexperienced by recurrent and distressing recollection and dreams of the event causing intense psychological distress and triggered by cues that symbolize or resemble the event. The individual will persistently avoid the stimuli associated with the trauma, but will have persistent symptoms of increased arousal, such as difficulty sleeping, irritability, difficulty with attention, increased vigilance, and exaggerated startle responses.

Generalized Anxiety Disorder (GAD)

GAD includes overanxious disorder of childhood. It is characterized by a general feeling of anxiety not tied to a specific event. The individual may have muscle tension, easy fatigability, irritability, restlessness, difficulty concentrating, and disturbed sleep.

Separation Anxiety Disorder (SAD)

SAD is typically a childhood disorder characterized by excessive anxiety when the child is separated from their home or the person to whom they are attached. The anxiety needs to be beyond what would be expected for the child's developmental level and the disturbance needs to last >4 weeks. It also must cause significant distress or impairment of function.

Obsessive-Compulsive Disorder (OCD)

OCD is characterized by persistent and recurring thoughts or impulses that are intrusive and inappropriate, and cause excessive anxiety. The individual tries to ignore or suppress the thoughts and realizes that they are created by their own mind or tries to neutralize them with other actions that become compulsions (repetitive behaviors, such as hand washing, that are repeated rigidly) in an attempt to reduce or prevent the distress. In cases in which there has been a sudden onset of OCD symptoms, the clinician should consider the possibility of pediatric autoimmune neuropsychiatric disorders associated with streptococcal infections (PANDAS).[22]

■ Motor Disorders and Physical Conditions

The three motoric disorders that can be commonly comorbid with ADHD are the two tic disorders, chronic tic disorder and Tourette's disorder, and the motor incoordination or dysfunction called developmental coordination disorder.

Tic/Tourette's Disorder

Tics are sudden, rapid, nonrhythmic, recurrent, and stereotyped motor or vocal movements that can cause marked distress. If they last for at least 4 weeks, but <1 year, the individual has a transient tic disorder. If they last for >12 months, but are all motor or all vocal, they constitute a chronic tic disorder, and if both motor and verbal tics are present for >1 year causing marked distress, this constitutes Tourette's disorder.

Developmental Coordination Disorder (DCD)

DCD is a marked impairment in motor coordination not due to a specific motor disorder such as cerebral palsy. Historically, it occurs in children who do poorly in athletic activities or fine-motor activities. On neurologic exam, the clinician can see difficulties in the child executing hand supination/pronation, finger-to-nose movements, crossing midline, and right/left identification. In children with severe incoordination, it is helpful to obtain an occupational therapy (OT) evaluation. If the child's handwriting is problematic, the OT evaluation may be provided by the school.

3

■ Physical Conditions

Some physical conditions are also associated with ADHD. Most individuals with generalized unresponsiveness to thyroid hormone (a relatively rare genetic disorder) also have ADHD, and many individuals who experience closed head injuries have behaviors compatible with ADHD. In addition, the effects of alcohol can cause ADHD symptoms as part of the fetal alcohol syndrome or with fetal alcohol effects, and ADHD symptoms can be seen in Fragile X syndrome, as mentioned previously.

REFERENCES

1. American Psychiatric Association. *Diagnostic and Statistical Manual of Mental Disorders, 4th ed, Text Revision*. Washington, DC: American Psychiatric Association; 2000.
2. Clinical practice guideline: diagnosis and evaluation of the child with attention-deficit/hyperactivity disorder. American Academy of Pediatrics. *Pediatrics*. 2000;105:1158-1170.
3. Smith BH, Pelham WE Jr, Gnagy E, Molina B, Evans S. The reliability, validity, and unique contributions of self-report by adolescents receiving treatment for attention-deficit/hyperactivity disorder. *J Consult Clin Psychol*. 2000;68:489-499.
4. Knouse LE, Bagwell CL, Barkley RA, Murphy KR. Accuracy of self-evaluation in adults with ADHD: evidence from a driving study. *J Atten Disord*. 2005;8:221-234.
5. Hoza B, Pelham WE Jr, Dobbs J, Owens JS, Pillow DR. Do boys with attention-deficit/hyperactivity disorder have positive illusory self-concepts? *J Abnorm Psychol*. 2002;111:268-278.
6. Mitsis EM, McKay KE, Schulz KP, Newcorn JH, Halperin JM. Parent-teacher concordance for DSM-IV attention-deficit/hyperactivity disorder in a clinic-referred sample. *J Am Acad Child Adolesc Psychiatry*. 2000;39:308-313.
7. Lahey B, Applegate B, Barkley RA, et al. DSM-IV field trials for oppositional defiant disorder and conduct disorder in children and adolescents. *Am J Psychiatry*. 1994;151:1163-1171.
8. Barkley RA, Murphy KR, Fischer M. *ADHD in Adults: What the Science Says*. New York, NY: Guilford Press; 2007.
9. Murphy K, Barkley RA. Prevalence of DSM-IV symptoms of ADHD in adult licensed drivers: implications for clinical diagnosis. *J Atten Disord*. 1996;1:147-161.
10. Danforth JS, DuPaul GJ. Interrater reliability of teacher rating scales for children with attention deficit hyperactivity disorder. *J Psychopathol Behav Assess*. 1996;18:227-237.
11. Wolraich ML, Drotar D, Felice M. *The Classification of Child and Adolescent Mental Conditions in Primary Care: Diagnostic and Statistical Manual for Primary Care (DSM-PC) Child and Adolescent Version*. Elk Grove, IL: American Academy of Pediatrics; 1996.
12. Wolraich ML, Feurer ID, Hannah JN, Baumgaertel A, Pinnock TY. Obtaining systematic teacher reports of disruptive behavior disorders utilizing DSM-IV. *J Abnorm Child Psychol*. 1998;26:141-152.
13. Swanson JM, Nolan W, Pelham WE. *SNAP Rating Scale*: Education Resources Information Center (ERIC); 1982.

14. DuPaul GJ, Power TJ, Anastopoulos AD, Reid R, McGoey KE, Ikeda MJ. Teacher ratings of attention deficit hyperactivity disorder symptoms: Factor structure and normative data. *Psychol Assess.* 1997;9:436-444.

15. Clinical practice guideline: diagnosis and evaluation of the child with attention-deficit/hyperactivity disorder. American Academy of Pediatrics. *Pediatrics.* 2000;105:1158-1170.

16. Conners C, Erhardt D, Sparrow EP. *CAARS-Self-Report: Long Version.* North Tonawanda, NY: Multi-Health Systems; 1997.

17. Kessler RC, Adler L, Ames M, et al. The World Health Organization Adult ADHD Self-Report Scale (ASRS): a short screening scale for use in the general population. *Psychol Med.* 2005;35:245-256.

18. Brown T. *Brown Attention-Deficit Disorder Scales.* San Antonio, CA: The Psychological Corporation; 1996.

19. McCann BS, Scheele L, Ward N, Roy-Byrne P. Discriminant validity of the Wender Utah Rating Scale for attention-deficit/hyperactivity disorder in adults. *J Neuropsychiatry Clin Neurosci.* 2000;12:240-245.

20. Gadow KD. Prevalence and efficacy of stimulant drug use with mentally retarded children and youth. *Psychopharmacol Bull.* 1985;21:291-303.

21. Aman MG, Marks RE, Turbott SH, Wilsher CP, Merry SN. Clinical effects of methylphenidate and thioridazine in intellectually subaverage children. *J Am Acad Child Adolesc Psychiatry.* 1991;30:246-256.

22. Swedo SE, Leonard HL, Garvey M, et al. Pediatric autoimmune neuropsychiatric disorders associated with streptococcal infections: clinical description of the first 50 cases. *Am J Psychiatry.* 1998;155:264-271.

4 Treating ADHD as a Chronic Illness

The approach to treating a patient with ADHD requires those same elements necessary in treating a patient with any chronic illness. ADHD is indeed a chronic illness because the available treatments address symptoms but are not curative, and the condition persists for at least an extended period of time, and in many patients, for their entire life. While some children are able to compensate well enough by adulthood, many continue to be symptomatic as adults. Fortunately, the available interventions are quite effective and most people with ADHD will be able to lead a successful life if treated appropriately. Therefore, ADHD meets all of the criteria for being a chronic condition, and it makes sense to use a chronic-care model in treating this condition.[1,2] This model includes the six elements presented in **Table 4.1**.

The first element refers to developing the necessary linkages to community resources, such as the school systems and mental health services. The second element refers to the extent to which medical services and the supporting organizations, such as health maintenance organizations, hospitals, and health insurers, are oriented to the model. Clinicians need to work with these organizations to collaborate in the chronic-care model approach. Self-management support refers to encouraging the patient and their family to become competent as the primary managers of the disorder. The more knowledgeable the patient (as he or she matures) and the family are about the condition, the more effective they will be in deciding on and following a treatment plan tailored to their preferences and needs. For children, it is also important to try to include the patient's teachers in the process. The fourth element refers to thinking of the practice as a system that includes nurses, receptionists, and billing staff, as well as consultants and other community staff providing services to the family as a team, and ensuring that the appropriate organizational and communication structures are in place.

TABLE 4.1 — Elements of a Chronic-Illness Approach to Treatment

• Community resources and policies
• Health care organization
• Self-management support
• Delivery system design
• Decision support
• Clinical information systems

It is important to establish links with mental health specialists when needed for the more complicated or difficult cases. It is best to develop a relationship with mental health consultants as part of practice procedures so that they are available when a patient with ADHD requires a referral. In many cases, the management plan may entail comanagement with therapy, such as parent management or coaching provided by the psychologist, while the primary care clinician manages the patient's medication. The more familiar the members of the team are with each other and the more effective their communication, the better they are able to meet the family's needs. Having an arrangement whereby the consultants are located in the same office or building has the advantage of easier communication between the families, the physician, and the consultants.

The fifth element, decision support, refers to ensuring that the clinician has access to current guidelines and the literature, and that there are consultants to provide optimal evidenced-based care. The last element, clinical information systems, refers to putting in place reminder systems to help monitor patients, to ensure adequate follow-up, and to provide feedback on how patients are performing on quality measures.

Developing a Management Plan for Patients With ADHD

A specific management plan should be developed collaboratively with the patient and their family, which should include a monitoring and follow-up process. In providing family and self-management support, it is helpful to encourage the patients and their parents to take an active role. It is very helpful to educate the families utilizing written, audio, and web-based materials and to encourage the families to connect to existing support groups. There should be a written treatment plan that has been developed collaboratively with the family. Follow-up and monitoring require defining target goals so that it is possible to identify progress. There needs to be a clear monitoring schedule for periodic follow-up, and in cases where the problems are too complicated to be easily addressed in a primary care setting, the clinician needs to work in conjunction with mental health specialists (including psychiatrists, psychologists, and other therapists). It is important to continue to monitor a patient's progress and to provide the continuity of a "medical home" even if the primary management of the mental health problems is shifted to a mental health clinician.[3] A suggested management plan is presented in **Figure 4.1**.

This plan can be modified to meet the needs of particular patients within the framework of the clinician's practice. The written plan should identify appropriate and achievable goals. The goals need to take into account the family's preferences, lifestyle, and culture. A process by which the goals can be periodically assessed with feedback from at least parents and teachers should be developed. The two therapies that have extensive research to support their efficacy are medications and behavior modification, which are discussed in Chapters 5 and 6. One of the difficulties in developing an appropriate treatment plan is that it is frequently difficult to receive the needed feedback, especially from teachers. This is even more difficult with preschool-age children in which case they may not have any observers other than the parent or may have a child-care worker with limited observational skills. The same holds true for adolescents who have multiple teachers who only see each student for a limited amount of time. Communication attempts are further hampered because participants in these discussions are rarely compensated for their time. The challenge can become even greater when there are inadequate mental health services to manage the difficult cases. Finally,

FIGURE 4.1 — ADHD Management Plan

Clinician

Name ____________________

Address ____________________

____

Telephone ____________________

Patient

Name ____________________

Date of Birth ____________________

School Name ____________________

School Telephone ____________________

Key Teacher Contact ____________________

Grade Level ____________________

Teacher E-mail Address or Fax ____________________

____

Diagnosis ____________________

____

____

Target Goals

1. ____________________
2. ____________________
3. ____________________

Treatment Plan

Medication ____________________

Dose ____________ Time ____________

Medication ____________________

Dose ____________ Time ____________

School Adjustments ____________________

____

____

Other Interventions ____________________

____

____

Strengths ____________________

____

____

Return Appointment ____________________

members of the popular press worsen the situation when they promote a negative image of the diagnosis and its treatment with stimulant medications.

To have a successful management plan requires good lines of communication between physicians, parents, children, their teachers, and, when needed, mental health consultants. To accomplish this goal, it is important to examine one's current office procedures in order to develop consistent and efficient methods of communication. Fax machines and the internet have improved both the ease and speed of communication. Use of rating scales, daily report cards (see Chapter 6, *Psychosocial Treatments*), and queries about target goals provided in written or electronic form can help to make communication more efficient.

4

All patients with ADHD need a basic understanding of the disorder. It is important to maintain confidentiality in this process. We have found that a critical issue to convey is that there is no association between ADHD and intelligence. We try to "destigmatize" ADHD by comparing it to having poor eyesight or having a chronic illness such as diabetes. In these conditions, the person is not at fault for having the disorder—they were born with it. They can be limited in life by the disorder unless it is treated, ie, with glasses or contacts or with medications. People who have these disorders recognize that they are not bad, damaged, or stupid—just someone who needs a bit of help in certain areas. It is the same with ADHD. Getting this point across can be challenging because a typical characteristic of individuals with ADHD is variable performance. A patient may have a good day when their attention is better than usual, followed by bad days when their attention is poorly focused. Teachers, parents, and other significant persons frequently come to the conclusion that if an individual can function well sometimes, the lack of function at other times is a willful choice. This observation is not correct because an individual's abilities will also be affected by a number of factors, such as their interest in the subject, extent of the distracters, and their mental and physical state at the time.

Approach With Adolescents

The path to maturity can be somewhat delayed in many young people with ADHD. In fact, a recent MRI study conducted at the National Institute of Mental Health (NIMH) documented that brain development occurred in a slightly delayed time frame in adolescents with ADHD in comparison with their non-ADHD peers.[4] In this study, the level of cortical thickening in those with ADHD reached the level of their peers at approximately 25 years of age. We know that ADHD does not usually disappear with the onset of adolescence or adulthood; however, those with ADHD continue to develop maturity over time and learn to compensate for the underlying neurologic deficits of ADHD. An important and often overlooked aspect of the care of young people with ADHD is the transition from adolescence to adulthood.

One of the important tasks of adolescence is to prepare for the responsibility of adulthood. Health care providers can play an active role in helping adolescents in this arena by gradually having them take on more responsibility and decision making as they get older. One way to begin this process is by giving young people a meaningful voice in their ADHD treatment from an early age. One of the authors (H.S.) typically states that there are three conditions under which medications will be used for ADHD:

- When the medication works well, ie, makes a significant difference in function
- When there are no significant side effects, ie, that the medication is very well tolerated
- Most important, when the patient agrees to a trial of medication.

This final condition begins in early adolescence so that the patient realizes that it is their choice whether they take medications. Obviously, one cannot force an adolescent to take medications, and the more they have the ability to make decisions for themselves, the more likely they are to be compliant with medications and develop the maturity that their parents hope they assume. Occasionally, an adolescent will clearly state that they do not want to take medications. In that situation, it is often useful to ask the adolescent what other measures they would like to take to improve their school, work, and social functioning. These may include increased motivation, working harder, tutoring, accommodations, counseling, parental involvement, etc. The goal is to create a partnership in which the adolescent feels their decisions are valued, and therefore, they are more likely to accept responsibility to the level they are capable. When given a clear choice, most often the adolescent will opt for a trial of medications. In addition, when deciding about the efficacy of medications and dosing levels that seem to be optimal, soliciting and acting upon the opinions of the adolescent are critical.

Another way to encourage the development of maturity is to start to see young people for part of their office visit alone, ie, without a parent or caregiver in the room. This can begin as early as at 11 to 12 years of age, but should certainly be a part of most office visits by the age of 14 or 15 years. Of course, the health care provider will be discussing the issue of confidential care and the limits of confidentiality with each adolescent as they begin to develop a relationship with their provider apart from their parents.

One of the important tasks of adolescence is to develop a stable sense of self and an identity as a competent and confident person. A simple method of encouraging the development of competence is to first identify areas in which the adolescent is already competent, such as sports, music, reading, math, video games, or artistic activities. It is important for adolescents to realize that they have learned certain skills. Next, one can inquire how they were able to acquire skills in this area. The answers will point out that there typically are ways that someone acquires skills: 1) they are interested in the area; 2) they practice the skills; and 3) they perform them. The clinician can then point out that they can acquire new skills and improve their performance in any area (most important, in school) by taking enough interest in the area to practice it (eg, doing their homework) and then by performing their new skills (eg, studying for tests and improving performance on them). In fact, it is clear that school performance is primarily dependent on simply doing homework, turning it in, and studying for tests. Encouraging an adolescent is often a matter of showing them that they are competent and that if they use skills they already have (eg, learning how to play a new video game or perfect a new dance or sports move), they can apply them to school work and improve their performance.

■ Driving

A major milestone in an adolescent's life is when they begin driving a car. This event immediately increases the risks of injuries due to motor vehicle accidents. It is well known in the insurance industry that adolescent drivers are more likely to have accidents than are adult drivers. In fact, the risk of accidents decreases with each year of driving experience gained until the age of approximately 25. Adolescents with ADHD have been shown to be poorer drivers than their non-ADHD peers. This fact should be emphasized with each family and careful decisions should be made on the restrictions regarding driving that will be applied to young ADHD drivers.[5] Preliminary studies have suggested that adolescents taking ADHD medications improve their driving skills.

■ Risk-Taking Behaviors

An area of importance to parents and health care providers of adolescents is risk-taking behaviors. These are likely to include experimentation with tobacco, alcohol, and possibly other drugs; sexuality-related behaviors; driving; and injury-related behaviors as well as other safety issues. All adolescents should be asked about their involvement in these areas at least once a year, as their answers are likely to change frequently as they grow and mature. An approach to these areas will be outlined in Chapter 8, *Substance Abuse Disorders and Issues Related to ADHD*, in a discussion on substance abuse and ADHD.

■ Planning for Independence

Because adolescents with ADHD are more likely to require help with organization, time management, decision making, homework, work, and other areas, parents and caregivers often develop patterns of careful monitoring and intervening on a regular basis in the affairs of the adolescent with ADHD. This is often necessary, but it may hamper the development of self-reliance skills in the adolescent. Therefore, when an adolescent is old enough to move away from home to attend college or work, they may not be ready to handle the responsibilities inherent in being more independent. Planning ahead as much as possible for this time is therefore important to try to assure a successful transition. During the high school years, we typically encourage parents to begin gradually and progressively to give more responsibility to their adolescents with ADHD.

The skills that they will need to acquire include how to negotiate academic establishments, perform laundry, handle bills and a bank account, budget finances, study effectively, plan study and writing time, cook, clean, and a variety of other life skills. The earlier they are able to learn those skills, the earlier they will be able to move away from home and begin an independent life.

When serious planning begins for the post–high school years, it is critical to do a careful evaluation of each adolescent with ADHD. The questions to address are presented in **Table 4.2**. College poses a number of challenges to the student with ADHD. Their schedules are likely to be considerably less regular than they have been in high school. Classes usually will not be daily and may occur only once a week. Assignments come due at variable times and require independent planning to complete in a timely fashion. In addition to these challenges, students often attend parties and participate in consuming alcohol and illegal substances. To address these challenges and choose the most appropriate environment with

TABLE 4.2 — Questions Pertaining to the Post–High School Adolescent With ADHD

- What setting will be best for them?
- Do they need to live at home for a year, work part-time, and go to a community college part-time?
- Should they live at home and attend a local 4-year university?
- Are they ready for an out-of-town or out-of-state college/university experience?

adequate support requires knowledge of the intelligence, skills, maturity, and responsibility of the individual. Precollege counseling should include a discussion of how the young person plans to handle these issues.

It is also important to help such students become comfortable with their diagnosis and knowledgeable about the condition so that they can become their own best advocate. Even in colleges with programs for students with ADHD, they may have to deal with professors who do not believe in the condition and inappropriately penalize students because of their condition. If students are planning to continue to take stimulant medication, they need to be warned about the risk of it being stolen or the risk of their getting in trouble with the authorities if they give away or sell their medication. We typically warn the patient that their medication could be harmful to others for whom a medical evaluation for clearance to take this medication has not been performed.

Choosing the right college for an ADHD adolescent can make the difference between academic success and failure. If the family and the adolescent choose a 4-year college/university, it is important to assess the type of experience they are likely to have. For example, large universities may offer less academic and personal support than a smaller college might offer. In addition, the family and the adolescent should carefully evaluate the office of student disabilities at prospective colleges or universities. Arranging a meeting with this office is an important part of any college visit. Representatives can give clear examples of the support and accommodations that are typically offered.

Individuals with ADHD are eligible for reasonable accommodations in both academic and vocational settings. In the United States, the Americans With Disabilities Act guarantees this right. Of course, for a young adult to take advantage of any accommodations, they must register with the Students With Disabilities Office at their school. To this end, their physician and/or psychologist should write a letter that confirms that this individual has been diagnosed with ADHD and suggest certain accommodations that seem reasonable. Such a letter usually suffices for accommodations at their school.

However, for accommodations for standardized testing, such as the ACT, SAT, MCAT, LSAT and GRE, a letter from a psychologist who has done extensive testing is usually necessary.

Young adults with ADHD who would like to choose a career in a branch of the armed services or the criminal justice department are faced with particular issues. The branches of the armed services are not required to follow the laws of the civilian sector with regard to disabilities and accommodations. Therefore, individuals with ADHD should expect that they will be treated no differently from any other recruit. In particular, they should not expect to be able to take ADHD medications. The regulations that the armed services use to determine who can be recruited change over time, but they typically do not allow individuals to apply who are on ADHD medications or who plan on taking them while in the service. On the other hand, the National Guard does not have such restrictions and individuals in the National Guard are able to continue to take ADHD medications while serving. Similarly, police and fire academies and departments are governed by civilian regulations and individuals may disclose that they have ADHD and then be allowed to take medications while studying and on the job. They will, of course, need to demonstrate that they are able to perform the job as well as other applicants.

Approach With Adults

After the diagnosis of ADHD is made in adults, the clinician should include several elements in a comprehensive management strategy. Ideally, this consists of education on ADHD, judicious and safe use of medications, and helping the patient identify and develop skills to compensate for the effects of the disorder. Education involves explaining that ADHD is primarily a heritable disorder, and it is not due to family situations or parenting practices. We briefly describe the research showing alterations in brain chemistry, neuroanatomy, and genetic alleles. It is explained that ADHD has no relationship to intelligence and is distributed widely in the population without regard to race, ethnicity, or socioeconomic status.

We explain to our patients that other mild disabilities commonly interfere with productivity in academic, employment, and social settings, and use the example we described for children regarding poor eyesight and the need for glasses. Many people have physical disorders, such as diabetes mellitus, which require ongoing medical therapy. ADHD is an analogous situation and therefore we attempt to destigmatize the disorder by comparison to other medical disorders. Finally, we recommend reading materials and web sites (such as www.chadd.org and www.adda.org) to help patients understand the disorder as much as possible.

Identification of any comorbidities is a critical step since most adults with ADHD will have at least one comorbid diagnosis, such as an anxiety disorder, an affective disorder, a substance-abuse disorder, or significant difficulties in their marriage or other relationships, or in their employment situation. Finally, a thorough medical evaluation should be done due to the increased medical comorbidities, such as hypertension, coronary heart disease, or cardiac arrhythmias.

Providing opportunities for patients and families to connect with other families is an important part of the education process. Other families frequently can provide practical advice as well as emotional support from having gone through a similar experience. Organized groups can also provide useful information and advocacy. There are two major national support organizations:

- Children and Adults With Attention Deficit Disorder, PO Box 2120, Hyattsville, MD 20748
- The National Attention-Deficit Disorders Association, 9930 Johnnycake Ridge, Suite 3E, Mentor, OH 44060.

These organizations have web sites that can be useful and informative to parents:

- CHADD (www.chadd.org)
- ADDA (www.add.org)
- ADD Warehouse 300 NW 70th, Suite 102, Plantation, FL 33317 (www.addwarehouse.com)
- National Institute for Mental Health (www.nimh.nih.gov/publicat/adhdmenu.cfm)

- Facts for Families (www.aacap.org)
- National Resource Center for ADHD (www.help 4adhd.org)

In communities with limited resources, the clinician may need to serve as a motivating and organizing force to help improve the community resources. These activities may include negotiating communication systems with the schools and clarifying the process about how children are assessed for educational problems. It can also include helping to establish a parent-support group or a parent-training program. As a respected member of the community, the clinician can be an effective motivating force.

4

REFERENCES

1. Bodenheimer T, Wagner EH, Grumbach K. Improving primary care for patients with chronic illness. *JAMA.* 2002;288:1775-1779.
2. Bodenheimer T, Wagner EH, Grumbach K. Improving primary care for patients with chronic illness: the chronic care model, Part 2. *JAMA*. 2002;288:1909-1914.
3. Medical Home Initiatives for Children With Special Needs Project Advisory Committee. American Academy of Pediatrics. The medical home. *Pediatrics*. 2002;110(1 Pt 1):184-186.
4. Shaw P, Eckstrand K, Sharp W, et al. Attention-deficit/hyperactivity disorder is characterized by a delay in cortical maturation. *Proc Natl Acad Sci USA*. 2007;104:19649-19654.
5. Barkley RA. Driving impairments in teens and adults with attention-deficit/hyperactivity disorder. *Psychiatr Clin North Am.* 2004;27:233-260.

5 Medication Treatment

FDA-Approved Medications

■ Stimulant Medications

History

Medication has been one of the mainstays of treating individuals with ADHD going back to the 1950s and 1960s when the condition was characterized as minimal brain damage. In fact, amphetamine as a treatment for behavioral disorders goes back to 1939 when Bradley reported appreciable behavioral improvement in children with behavioral disorders who were given Benzedrine to treat headaches that were caused by lumbar punctures required to perform pneumoencephalograms.[1]

Despite Bradley's article, clinical use did not start in earnest until 10 to 20 years later, initially with dextroamphetamine and subsequently with methylphenidate. These two medications went through extensive studies in the 1970s and 1980s and continue to be the first line of medication treatment for ADHD. Because the effects of the medications were of short duration, lasting 4 to 5 hours, they required administration 2 to 4 times a day. Attempts to find longer-lasting or alternative treatments led initially to the development of a wax matrix methylphenidate compound (Ritalin SR) and a dextroamphetamine spansule (Dexedrine Spansules) to extend the duration of action of these short-acting preparations. The initial long-acting formulations were limited in extending the duration of effects, likely because they did not take into consideration the need for the more rapid rise occurring with the immediate-release form and the need for a continued rise in blood levels to sustain the effects as demonstrated in **Figure 5.1**.[2]

Other alternative medications, such as pemoline or tricyclic antidepressants, were also found to be efficacious, but they were more likely to have significant side effects or narrower margins of safety.

FIGURE 5.1 — Blood Concentration of Methylphenidate Over Time

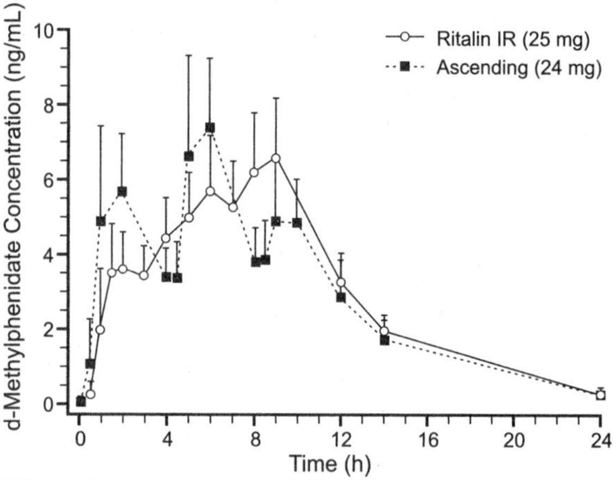

The changes in blood level over time between immediate release given three times a day and OROS methylphenidate given once a day.

Swanson JM, et al. *J Am Acad Child Adolesc Psychiatry*. 2002;41: 1306-1314.

Evidence of Efficacy

The stimulant medications (dextroamphetamine, mixed amphetamine salts, dexamphetamine, and methylphenidate) are the most studied psychotropic medications. There have been >300 studies in >6000 subjects demonstrating their short-term efficacy. The majority of research has studied the effects of methylphenidate on elementary school–aged children. With appropriate titration, approximately 70% will respond to the first stimulant medication with which they are treated. If those who do not respond are systematically tried on a second stimulant medication in the same manner, a total of approximately 80% to 90% will respond. There are far fewer studies in adolescents and adults, but the response rates have been similar to those achieved in children.[3,4]

While dextroamphetamine is approved for use in children as young as 3 years of age, and methylphenidate is only approved for children 6 years and older, these decisions reflect the particular circumstances in which the medication was approved rather than clear differences in scientific evidence. In preschool-age children, the majority of the studies have examined methylphenidate. The largest and most recent study was a multisite study that found methylphenidate to be safe and effective in 4- to 5-year-old children with ADHD.[5] However, it found children to have slower metabolic rates so that lower doses and longer durations per dose are required. The dose-response curve from that study is shown in **Figure 5.2**. In addition, side effects were seen more frequently. As seen in older children, some degree of growth suppression was observed. The expected growth potential of the child and the family's concern about their child's height are important to consider when deciding to start treatment and it is critical to closely monitor height. It may also be more difficult to establish the diagnosis in preschool children, and there is the theoretic concern about starting a CNS medication while the brain is in an earlier stage of development. Therefore, for preschool

5

FIGURE 5.2 — Methylphenidate Dose Response: Efficacy From Crossover Phase Indicating Improvement in ADHD Symptoms With Increased Dose

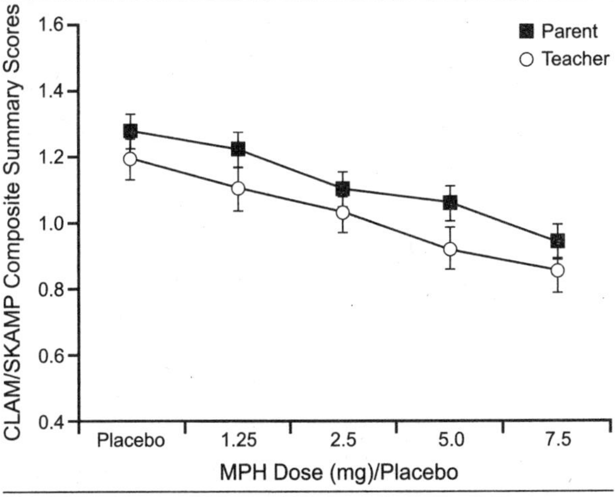

Adapted from: Greenhill L, et al. *J Am Acad Child Adolesc Psychiatry.* 2006;45:1284-1293.

children, it is best to use the cautious approach employed in the multisite study.[6] They first asked families to participate in a behavior-based parent-training program for 14 weeks and only started medication in those children whose behavior was not significantly improved by the parenting program. For one third of the families enrolled, the behavioral intervention was sufficient to improve their child's behavior. Some of these children may subsequently require medication, but the intervention was able to delay its introduction to an older age when the risks and benefits are better defined.

In adolescents and adults, the studies show effects similar to those seen in children. As with very small children, it may be somewhat more difficult to diagnose ADHD in adolescents if it is not diagnosed at a younger age, and there is a similarly rapid growth of the brain during this time.[7] In addition, adolescents may be less likely to accept medication therapy and therefore one should include them in the discussion about whether to start medication. The effects of medication therapy are similar in adolescents to those in younger children, as are the choice of medication and the dose utilized. Adolescents and adults with ADHD are more likely to have comorbid conditions, such as depressive, anxiety, bipolar, and substance-use disorders (SUDs). In these situations, the choice of medication may be altered by the comorbid conditions.[8,9]

The stimulant medications reduce the core symptoms of inattention, hyperactivity, and impulsivity. They also improve academic productivity, although they do not improve cognitive abilities or academic performance. Furthermore, in some children, they will reduce oppositional and aggressive behaviors, and impulsive and delinquent behaviors in some adolescents and adults. It is helpful to measure medications by determining their impact on the patient's core symptoms. These symptoms are most likely to show a noticeable change in response to medication and are likely to be the cause of impairment in a patient with ADHD.[10]

While the evidence for the short-term efficacy of stimulant medications is quite clear, the evidence for long-term efficacy is not as clear.[11] Evidence from the NIMH

Multi-Modal Therapy of ADHD (MTA) trial supports efficacy for at least 36 months, although it is variable across patients, and the longer-term studies suggest improvement but are less well designed.[12] Longer-term studies in preschoolers, adolescents, and adults are lacking.

The five stimulant medications, dextroamphetamine, methylphenidate, dexmethylphenidate, lisdexamfetamine, and mixed amphetamine salts, have similar effects, side effects, and safety profiles. However, there are differences in plasma curves and duration of action, dependent on the delivery systems of the medications. In addition, while methylphenidate may lower the seizure threshold and dextroamphetamine does not, both medications have been used to treat children with ADHD and seizure disorders with no recurrence of seizures as long as the seizure disorder is adequately controlled. Even in individuals with other comorbid conditions, such as anxiety or mood disorders, it is generally preferable to first treat the ADHD with stimulant medications if the comorbid conditions are mild because the mood or anxiety symptoms may diminish significantly if the stress caused by the ADHD is reduced. In those instances in which the mood or anxiety disorder is severe and is causing a great deal of symptoms, it may be preferable to initiate therapy with a medication for these symptoms prior to starting a stimulant medication.

Misconceptions

There are several misconceptions about stimulant medications. The effects of the medications are not paradoxical, ie, the reason that individuals with ADHD seem calmer and more focused when taking a stimulant medication is due to the fact that the medication is ameliorating the underlying core ADHD symptoms. Stimulant medications act as dopamine and norepinephrine agonists that block their reuptake, primarily in the caudate nucleus and prefrontal cortex. It is generally accepted that the pathophysiologic basis of ADHD is a relative deficiency of dopamine and norepinephrine in those areas of the brain.

Second, a response to medication cannot be used as a diagnostic test for ADHD. Since stimulants can improve performance in a variety of areas, individuals without ADHD may also see improved performance. Conversely, if an individual does not respond to a stimulant, it does not rule out the diagnosis of ADHD, since a minority of those individuals with ADHD will not respond to medication. Children, adolescents, and adults who are treated for ADHD usually do not find stimulant medications pleasurable and do not commonly abuse them. In individuals who do abuse stimulant medications, they usually have to take the medications intranasally or intravenously to obtain the euphoric feeling they seek. Several of the new formulations of stimulants are less likely to be abused via these routes, such as OROS-methylphenidate (Concerta), methylphenidate patch (Daytrana), and lisdexamfetamine (Vyvanse). They also usually require doses that are 10 to 100 times the dose recommended for treating individuals with ADHD.

Titration

With appropriate titration, approximately 70% will respond to whichever stimulant medication is chosen for initial therapy. While patients will vary in their response to the initial therapy both with regard to efficacy and adverse effects, it is not possible to predict the response of each individual patient. Therefore, the choice of starting with either a methylphenidate or amphetamine product is primarily dependent on the personal preferences of the family and their clinician. If the response to the initially chosen medication is determined not to be beneficial after an adequate trial, it is useful to try the alternative group (methylphenidate vs amphetamine).

The clinical response to stimulants is not related to weight or any other identifiable characteristics. Therefore, it is most useful to titrate the medication systematically at first, starting at the lowest dose and titrating up until attaining a maximal effect or causing significant adverse effects. If the maximal dose is attained without appreciable improvement in the core symptoms, it is then useful to try a medication from the alternative stimulant medication group in the same manner. In this way, a total of approximately 80% to 90% will respond to one of the stimulants.[12] While it has not been substantiated in controlled studies, clinical experience suggests that some patients may need doses that are above the maximal doses listed in the package insert, which should be carefully titrated while monitoring for any adverse effects.

A listing of the stimulant medications and their dosages and pharmacokinetics is shown in **Table 5.1**.

Methylphenidate

Methylphenidate is a piperidine derivative that is a racemic compound. The levo isomer is rapidly metabolized and essentially inactive. Short-acting methylphenidate has a half-life of 2 to 3 hours and duration of action of approximately 4 hours. Liquid and chewable forms are now available for patients who have difficulty swallowing tablets or capsules.

5

Efron and coworkers compared the efficacy of immediate-release methylphenidate (0.3 mg/kg twice daily) and immediate-release dexamphetamine (0.15 mg/kg twice daily) in a 2-week, double-blind, crossover study in 125 children with ADHD.[13] Outcome measures included Conners' Parent Rating Scale-Revised (CPRS-R), Conners' Teacher Rating Scale-Revised (CTRS-R), and a Parent Global Perceptions questionnaire.

Treatment with both stimulants resulted in significant group mean improvements from baseline score on all measures, although the CTRS-R response was greater with methylphenidate on the conduct problems and hyperactivity factors, as well as on the hyperactivity index. On the CPRS-R, anxiety was the only factor to differ significantly in favor of methylphenidate. Parents rated 73% of subjects as globally improved on methylphenidate and 69% improved on dexamphetamine compared with baseline. Overall, 46% of parents chose methylphenidate as the preferred drug compared with 37% who chose dexamphetamine. As shown in **Table 5.2**, the proportion of patients who were considered responders to each of the two stimulants did not differ significantly, although the responder rates varied according to the assessment criteria. The data presented in **Table 5.3** address the important clinical question "If a child does not respond to one stimulant, what is the likelihood of response to the alternative stimulant?" Again, the

TABLE 5.1 — Stimulant Medications: Dosing and Pharmacokinetics

Generic Compounds	Brand Names	Starting Dose (mg)	Dosing Frequency	Duration of Action (hr)	Max Dose (mg)	Available Formulations and Doses (mg)
Mixed amphetamine salts	Adderall	2.5-5	qd-bid	6	40	Tablets: 5, 7.5, 10, 12.5, 15, 20, 30
	Adderall XR	10	qd	10-12	40	Capsules: 5, 10, 15, 20, 25, 30
Dextroamphetamine	Dexedrine	2.5	bid-tid	4-6	40	Tablets: 5
	Dexedrine Spansule	5	qd-bid	6+	40	Capsules: 5, 10, 15
	Dextrostat	2.5	bid-tid	4-6	40	Tablets: 5, 10
Lisdexamfetamine	Vyvanse	20	qd	12	70	Capsules: 20, 30, 40, 50, 60, 70
Methylphenidate	Concerta	18	qd	12	54	Capsules: 18, 27, 36, 54
	Daytrana	10	Apply for 9 hr	11-12	30	Patches: 10, 15, 20, 30
	Metadate CD	20	qd	6-8	60	Capsules: 10, 20, 30, 40, 50, 60
	Methylin	5	bid-tid	3-5	60	Tablets: 5,10, 20
	Methylin ER	5	bid-tid	3-5	60	Tablets: 10, 20
	Ritalin	5	bid-tid	3-5	60	Tablets: 5, 10, 20
	Ritalin LA	20	qd	6-8	60	Capsules: 10, 20, 30, 40
	Ritalin SR	20	qd-bid	2-6	60	Tablets: 20
Dexmethylphenidate	Focalin	2.5	bid	3-5	40	Tablets: 2.5, 5, 10
	Focalin XR	5	qd	8-12	20	Capsules: 5, 10, 15, 20

TABLE 5.2 — Proportion of Responders and Nonresponders to DEX[a] and MPH[a]

	Responders to…			Nonresponders to	
Measure	Both (%)	DEX but not MPH (%)	MPH but not DEX (%)	Both (%)	*P* value
Parent global perceptions	46.4	21.6	25.6	5.6	0.60
CPRS-R (hyperactivity)	57.6	16.8	15.2	8.0	0.87
CTRS-R (hyperactivity)	41.6	12.8	20.0	20.0	0.21

[a] Immediate-release formulation.

Adapted from: Efron D, et al. *Pediatrics*. 1997;100:1-7.

TABLE 5.3 — Proportion of Nonresponders to One Stimulant Who Responded to the Other Stimulant

Measure	Nonresponders to DEX[a] (%)	DEX[a] Nonresponders Who Responded to MPH[a] (%)	Nonresponders to MPH[a] (%)	MPH[a] Nonresponders Who Responded to DEX[a] (%)
Parent global perceptions	31.2	82.0	27.2	79.4
CPRS-R (hyperactivity)	23.2	65.5	24.8	67.7
CTRS-R (hyperactivity)	40.0	50.0	32.8	39.0

[a] Immediate-release formulation.

Adapted from: Efron D, et al. *Pediatrics*. 1997;100:1-7.

proportions of nonresponders to one agent who responded to the alternate stimulant were similar, although the rates varied according to the criteria.

Within the past several years, there has been an increase in the number of delivery systems available to administer methylphenidate. The new delivery systems help to extend the duration of action of the medication. The purpose of extending the duration is to reduce the frequency of doses required for treatment and, particularly, to avoid having to administer the medication at school. The oldest compound is methylphenidate sustained release (Ritalin SR). The extension of the duration of action of this delivery system has been less than initially expected. It generally lasts approximately 5 hours.

A newly improved system that utilizes microbead technology (intermediate-release methylphenidate—Metadate CD or Ritalin LA) has extended the duration to 8 hours (equivalent to twice-a-day dosing of regular methylphenidate). Both Metadate CD and Ritalin LA employ microbead controlled-release technology to mimic twice-daily administration of methylphenidate. However, they primarily vary in the ratio of immediate-release and extended-release beads: 50/50 immediate- to extended-release beads in Ritalin LA and a 30/70 ratio in Metadate CD. Therefore, patients requiring a larger immediate response will respond better to Ritalin LA, while those requiring more in the afternoon will respond better to Metadate CD.

The efficacy of methylphenidate CD (Metadate CD) was compared with placebo in a 3-week, randomized, double-blind, crossover trial in 314 children and adolescents 6 to 16 years of age with ADHD in a community setting in which a single teacher could make behavioral assessments in the morning and afternoon.[14] Following a 1-week, single-blind, placebo-washout period, patients were treated for 3 weeks with methylphenidate CD titrated to efficacy and tolerability (mean dose 40.7 mg/day) or placebo. The primary efficacy variable was the Connors' Teacher Global Index (CTGI). After 1, 2, and 3 weeks of treatment, CTGI scores were significantly reduced from baseline with methylphenidate CD treatment ($P=0.0001$) vs placebo treatment (**Figure 5.3**).

FIGURE 5.3 — Effect of Metadate CD and Placebo on CTGI Scores in Children and Adolescents Treated in a Community Classroom Setting

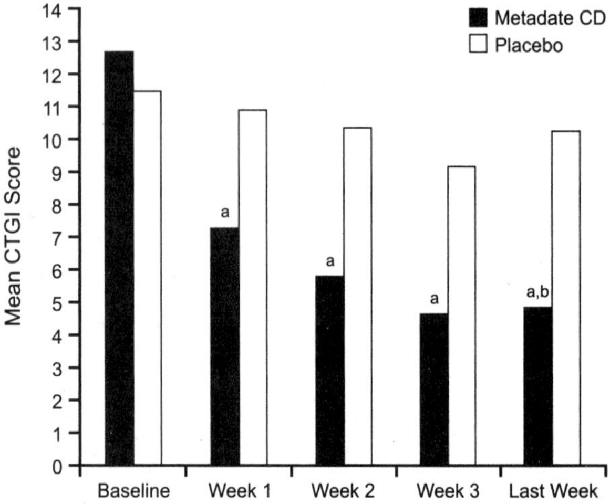

[a] P=0.0001 vs placebo.
[b] P<0.05 vs baseline.

Anderson VR, Keating GM. *Pediatr Drugs*. 2006;8:319-333.

"Last-week" analysis (average of all individual morning and afternoon assessments from each of 3 observation days in the third week of treatment) indicated that CTGI scores also were significantly (P <0.05) reduced from baseline in methylphenidate CD–treated patients but not in those who received placebo.

Biederman and associates compared the efficacy and safety of Ritalin LA in a randomized, parallel-group, placebo-controlled study in children with ADHD aged 6 to 14 years.[15] Following titration and a 1-week placebo washout period, patients were randomized to 2 weeks of double-blind treatment with either Ritalin LA or placebo. Efficacy was assessed by change from baseline (end of placebo washout) in Connors' ADHD/*DSM-IV* Rating Scale for Teachers (CADS-T) total and Inattention and Hyperactivity/Impulsivity subscale scores and the ADHD/*DSM-IV* rating scale for Parents (CADS-P) total and subscale scores. In the 134 responders included in the intent-to-treat analysis, those treated with Ritalin LA exhibited a significantly greater improvement than those treated with placebo in the CADS-T total score (–10.7 vs 2.8, respectively; P <0.0001) and significantly greater improvements in the CADS Inattention and Hyperactivity/ Impulsivity subscales. There also were significant treatment differences in change from baseline in the three CADS-P subscales (**Figure 5.4**).

Unlike Metadate CD and Ritalin LA, which employ microbead technology, OROS methylphenidate (Concerta) uses an osmotic pump mechanism and has the greatest extended duration of action of 12 hours. Its capsule does not dissolve in the gastrointestinal (GI) system, therefore, it is contraindicated in patients who have any significant constrictures in the GI tract.

5

A 28-day, randomized, parallel-group, double-blind trial in 282 children 6 to 12 years of age with ADHD assessed the efficacy and tolerability of once-daily OROS methylphenidate, three-times daily immediate-release (IR) methylphenidate dosed every 4 hours, and placebo.[16] As shown in **Figure 5.5**, the results of the primary efficacy measure, the teacher IOWA Conners I/O subscale

FIGURE 5.4 — Mean Changes From Baseline in CADS-P Total and Subscale Scores After 2-Weeks' Treatment With Ritalin LA or Placebo

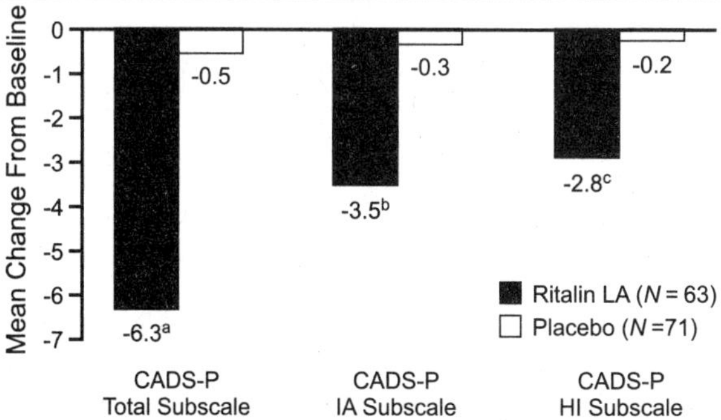

[a] P<0.00043.
[b] P<0.0213.
[c] P<0.0015 vs placebo.

Adapted from: Beiderman J, et al. *Pediatr Drugs*. 2003;5:833-841.

FIGURE 5.5 — Teacher IOWA Conners I/O Scores in Children With ADHD Treated With OROS MPH, IR MPH, or Placebo

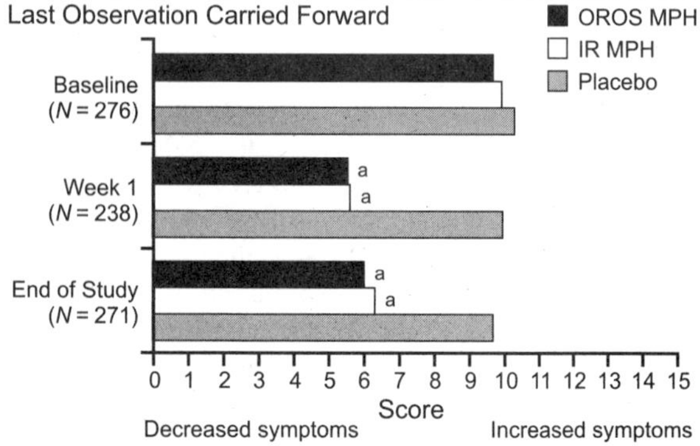

[a] P<0.001 vs placebo.

Adapted from: Wolraich ML, et al. *Pediatrics*. 2001;108:883-892.

completed at end of study, showed that both OROS methylphenidate (mean: 5.98 ± 3.91) and IR methylphenidate (mean: 6.35 ± 4.31) were significantly better (P <0.001) than placebo (mean: 9.77 ± 4.02). However, there was no significant difference between the mean IOWA Conners scores for the OROS methylphenidate and IR methylphenidate treatment groups at week 1 or at the end of the study. Teacher and parent SNAP-IV scores evaluating inattention, hyperactivity/impulsivity, and ODD behaviors were also significantly better (P <0 .001) in patients who were in the active-treatment groups. There was no significant difference between these measures in the two active-treatment groups.

OROS methylphenidate was recently approved for the treatment of adults with ADHD. The efficacy and safety of OROS methylphenidate in adults was demonstrated in a 6-week, randomized, placebo-controlled trial in 141 adults with *DSM-IV* ADHD.[4] Compared with placebo, treatment with OROS methylphenidate resulted in significant improvement in *DSM-IV* symptoms of inattention (P <0.001) and hyperactivity/impulsivity (P=0.03) (**Figure 5.6**).

FIGURE 5.6 — Change in *DSM-IV* Symptom Clusters After 6-Weeks' Treatment With OROS Methylphenidate in Adults With ADHD

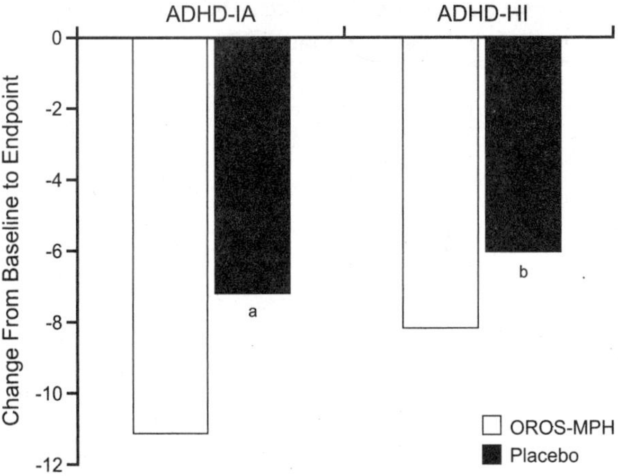

[a] $P < 0.001$.
[b] $P = 0.03$.

Biederman J, et al. *Biol Psychiatry*. 2006;59:829-835.

Dexmethylphenidate (Focalin) is a compound that contains only the pharmacologically active dexmethylphenidate. There is also an extended-release dexmethylphenidate (Focalin XR) utilizing the microbead technology in a 50/50 mixture of immediate- and extended-release beads, but it appears to have a longer extended-release time, in some cases up to 12 hours.

The extended-bead–release systems allow for the capsules to be opened and the beads sprinkled on food for those patients who have difficulty swallowing capsules.

A recent multicenter, double-blind, crossover study compared the efficacy of extended-release dexmethylphenidate with extended-release *d,l*-methylphenidate and placebo in children 6 to 12 years of age in a laboratory classroom setting.[17] The primary efficacy endpoint was change from baseline on the SKAMP rating scale combined score (**Figure 5.7**). Both extended-release dexmethylphenidate and extended-release *d,l*-methylphenidate were signifi-

FIGURE 5.7 — Adjusted Mean Changes From Predose in SKAMP Combined Scores in Children With ADHD Using Extended-Release Dexmethylphenidate, Extended-Release *d,l*-methylphenidate, or Placebo

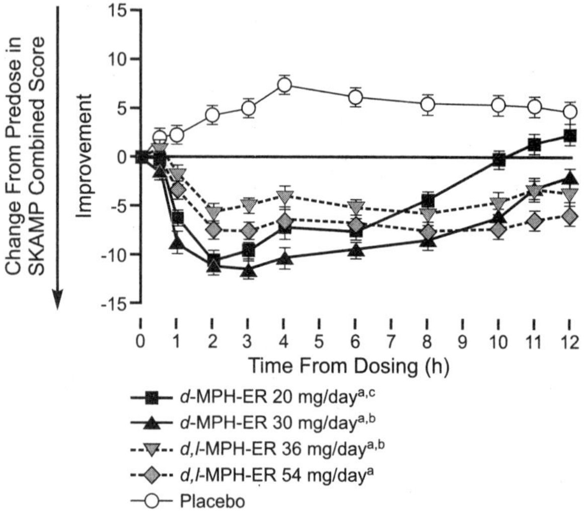

[a] $P<0.001$ vs placebo: *d*-MPH-ER 20 mg/day 1-10 hours post-dose; *d*-MPH-ER 30 mg/day 1-12 hours postdose; *d,l*-MPH-ER 36 mg/day 2-12 hours postdose; *d,l*-MPH-ER 54 mg/day 1-12 hours postdose.
[b] $P=0.001$ vs placebo: *d*-MPH-ER 30 mg/day 0.5 hours post-dose; *d,l*-MPH-ER 36 mg/day 1 hour postdose.
[c] $P<0.05$ vs placebo: *d*-MPH-ER 20 mg/day 0.5 and 11 hours postdose.

Adapted from: Muniz R, et al. *J Child Adolesc Psychopharmacol.* 2008;18:248-256.

cantly superior to placebo at all time points during the study with the exception of 20 mg/day extended-release dexmethylphenidate at 12 hours postdose.

A dermal methylphenidate patch (Daytrana) also is able to provide extended effects for up to 12 hours. The duration can be tailored to the patient's needs by removing the patch sooner than the 9 hours recommended for providing a 12-hour duration. It is important to note that the actual duration of action for any of these medications will vary from patient to patient. The dermal methylphenidate patch was compared with a placebo patch in 80 children aged 6 to 12 years with a *DSM-IV* diagnosis of ADHD in a randomized, crossover, analogue classroom study.[18] At all individual postdose time points measured, mean SKAMP-D scores were significantly lower (improved) with MTS treatment than with placebo treatment. The difference was statistically significant ($P < 0.01$) beginning with the first postdose assessment at 2 hours and continuing throughout the laboratory classroom day to include the final postdose assessment at 12 hours (**Figure 5.8**). Analysis of SKAMP Attention (SKAMP-A) subscale scores showed similar statistically significant results ($P < 0.0001$).

5

The most common side effects of methylphenidate are decreased appetite, sleep disturbance, and headache. The appetite will frequently increase after several months. If the patient's weight is affected, use of calorie-enriched food may be helpful. It is important to determine the patient's current and past history of sleep and headache.

FIGURE 5.8 — Mean SKAMP-D Subscale Scores by Time Point in Children Age 6 to 12 Years With ADHD: Methylphenidate Transdermal System vs Placebo

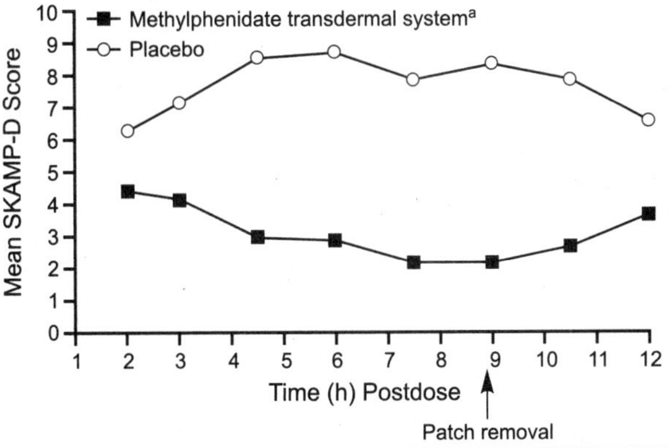

[a] $P < 0.01$ at all points for methylphenidate transdermal system compared with placebo using ANOVA.

Adapted from: McGough JJ, et al. *J Attention Disord.* 2006;9:476-485.

Sleep problems are frequently present in patients with ADHD independent of their treatments. When patients are overly sensitive to the medication or when they are given too high a dose, they may develop psychotic symptoms (rarely) or become overfocused (commonly). These side effects can sometimes be resolved with lowering the dose. Overfocusing usually manifests by the patient becoming listless, or what parents refer to as "appearing like a zombie." The usual course of tics and tic disorders is for the tics to wax and wane. This pattern can make it difficult to determine whether there is a relationship between the methylphenidate and the tics. If children have tics and require methylphenidate, in approximately one third there will be an increase in the tics, in approximately one third there will be a decrease in the tics, and in approximately one third the medication will have no effect on the tics.[19]

Some children will have a decrease in their rate of growth. There have been conflicting data as to whether there is catch-up growth once the medications are stopped and if medication holidays are beneficial. It is important to discuss this potential side effect with patients and families and to carefully monitor the patient's growth.

Because the response of stimulant medication is so variable from patient to patient, doses related to the size of the patient (mg/kg) are not as relevant as they are in pediatric patients for other medications. The most appropriate process is to start at the lowest dose (5 mg/dose for methylphenidate or 2.5 mg/dose in children <5 years of age) and gradually increase the dose until the optimal dose is achieved with the least side effects, up to the maximum dose of 60 mg/day or 20 mg/dose of IR formulations. Some patients may require a higher dose than the Food and Drug Administration (FDA)–approved 60-mg/day dose, but it is important to note this is not within the FDA-approved range, is not based on empiric evidence, and requires careful monitoring to identify patients who develop tolerance to the medications. The IR methylphenidate preparations can be given twice or three times a day based on the patient's need for symptomatic relief and the family's preferences. Intermediate- and extended-release preparations are generally given once a day, making administration easier for parents and patients.

However, if a more extended time is required, the 8-hour preparations require an additional IR formulation to be given in the afternoon in order to cover the rest of the day. This treatment plan can enable the use of a reduced afternoon dose in situations where an extended-release preparation causes an increase in sleep difficulties. Some patients only require coverage for 8 hours. For example, those patients with the inattentive subtype that is primarily creating school dysfunction may get by with morning and noontime dosing or one dose of an 8-hour preparation, while patients with the combined type are more likely to require tid dosing or a 12-hour extended-release preparation because they are dysfunctional at both school and home. Adolescents and adults may require longer durations of action and therefore may occasionally need to have extended-release preparations given twice a day. 5

The new extended-release formulations all have some IR components. For OROS methylphenidate (Concerta), the equivalent of 10 mg methylphenidate TID is 36 mg, and it has 8-mg IR. For Ritalin LA or dexmethylphenidate (Focalin XR), the ratio of immediate- to extended-release is 50/50, so the 20-mg capsules, which are equivalent to 10 mg bid, have 10 mg IR. Metadate CD, with a 30/70 ratio, has 6 mg IR. **Figure 5.9** indicates

FIGURE 5.9 — Duration of Action of Methylphenidate Products

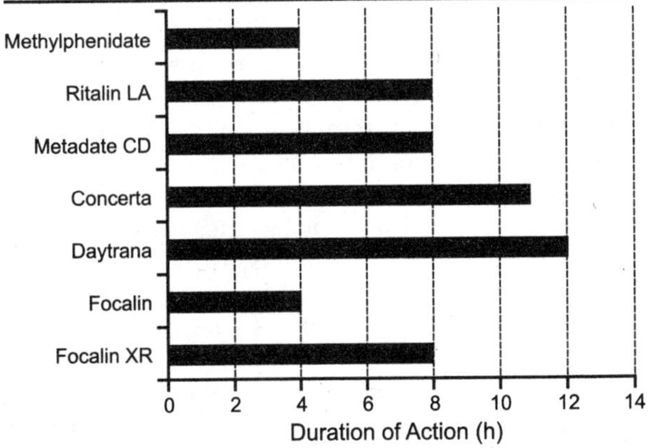

the average duration of action, although the duration is likely to vary for individual patients.

While obtaining a complete blood count periodically is in the original instructions for the prescription of methylphenidate, it has not been found to be needed, and no specific laboratory assessments are required. Since the blood levels do not correlate well with behavioral changes, they are also of little clinical use.

Recently, a great deal of attention has been devoted to the potential for serious cardiac side effects of stimulant therapy. In 2005, Adderall was taken off the market in Canada for several months because of this concern. The FDA convened a panel to examine the issue of stimulants and cardiovascular safety. Sudden cardiac death (SCD) occurred in approximately 0.2-0.4 children and adolescents taking stimulants per 100,000 patient years. Most of these children had underlying congenital heart disorders, such as hypertrophic cardiomyopathy (HC). Since the background prevalence of SCD in children (1.5-8.3 per 100,000 patient years) is actually higher than that observed in children on stimulants, there seems to be a very small risk that stimulants are a primary factor in these deaths.[20]

Nevertheless, it is clear that stimulants should not be prescribed for a patient with serious underlying cardiac disorders without a full cardiac evaluation. Therefore, careful screening for family histories of early myocardial infarctions, serious arrhythmias, congenital cardiac defects (especially HC), and SCD is mandatory. The health care provider should also ask about a personal history of heart disease, hypertension, heart murmur, palpitations and arrhythmias, syncope, dizziness on exertion, chest discomfort, and shortness of breath. A cardiac work-up should be undertaken in any patient with a history or physical exam findings suggestive of risk for cardiac disease. This evaluation is critical and a reason why primary care physicians are in an excellent position to become the primary providers for adult patients with ADHD.

The American Heart Association (AHA) has recently recommended both the screening outlined above to elicit a history of cardiac disease and a physical examination, as well as obtaining an electrocardiogram (ECG) because of the very rare cases of sudden death found in postmarketing surveillance.[21] However, it is not clear that individuals being treated with stimulant medications are at any increased risk over the population in general, as the rates of SCD in children not taking stimulant medications are greater than rates calculated for those children taking such medications. While episodes of SCD are obviously devastating, they are extremely rare so that the cost and difficulty of obtaining ECGs and the effects of false-positives are reasons why the recommendations of the AHA were not supported by the American Academy of Pediatrics (AAP) or the American Academy of Child and Adolescent Psychiatry (AACAP).[22] The statement has been jointly revised by the AHA, AAP, and AACAP and now states that an ECG is not mandatory but optional at the discretion of the physician.[23]

In addition to the careful family and personal history outlined above, a cardiac examination and monitoring of blood pressure and heart rate should be undertaken. Abnormal findings should be fully assessed and a referral to a cardiologist should be considered before starting a patient on stimulant medications.

Amphetamines

The profile of action and side effects for amphetamines is very similar to that of methylphenidate. Short-acting dextroamphetamine has a half-life of 4 to 6 hours and a duration of action of approximately 5 hours, while other amphetamine formulations have a longer duration of action. **Figure 5.10** provides the average duration of action for each of the amphetamine medications, although the actual length will vary with each individual.

Like methylphenidate, the most common side effects are anorexia, sleep disturbance, and headache. The appetite will frequently increase after several months. Height also needs to be monitored closely. If the patient's weight is affected, use of calorie-enriched food may be helpful. It is important to determine the patient's current and past history of sleep and headache. Sleep problems are frequently present in patients with ADHD, independent of their treatments.

FIGURE 5.10 — Duration of Action of Amphetamine Products

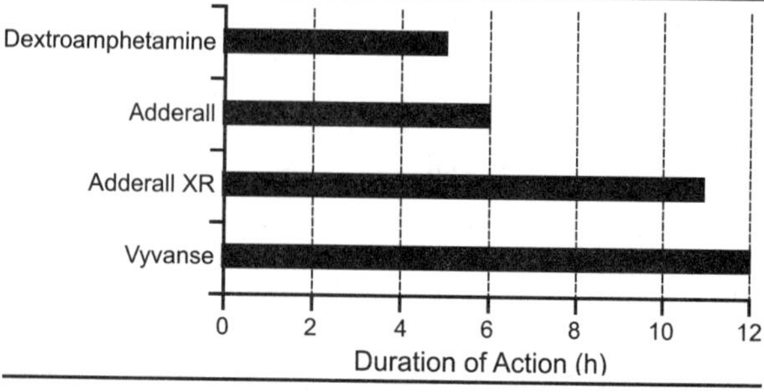

As with methylphenidate, in patients who are overly sensitive or when the dose is too high, patients may rarely develop psychotic symptoms or become overfocused. The overfocusing side effect can usually be resolved with lowering the dose. Overfocusing usually manifests by the patient becoming listless (ie, appearing "like a zombie"). The usual course of tics and tic disorders is for the tics to wax and wane. This pattern can make it difficult to determine the relationship between the dextroamphetamine and the tics. The side effects profile of methylphenidate and that of amphetamines are essentially the same, with the exception of several minor differences. There is more appetite suppression with dextroamphetamine, and dextroamphetamine does not lower the seizure threshold, while methylphenidate does slightly.

Like methylphenidate, because the response of stimulant medication is so variable from patient to patient, doses related to the size of the patient (mg/kg) are not as relevant in pediatric patients as they are for other medications. The most appropriate process is to start at the lowest dose (5 mg/dose or 2.5 mg/dose in children <5 years of age) and gradually increase the dose until the optimal dose is achieved with the least side effects, with the maximum dose being 40 mg/day. The dextroamphetamine can be given two or three times a day based on the patient's need for symptomatic relief and the family's preferences. It has a slightly longer duration of action than methylphenidate. As with methylphenidate, no laboratory tests need to be monitored and blood levels are not of clinical utility. The same issue discussed previously about obtaining ECGs for children treated with methylphenidate also pertains to amphetamines.

Mixed Amphetamine Salts

Mixed amphetamine salts (Adderall) are a mixture of 75% dextroamphetamine and 25% levo-amphetamine. Unlike methylphenidate, both the dextro and levo forms of amphetamine are pharmacologically active. It appears to have a longer duration of action than methylphenidate, but it has never been assessed in direct comparison to dextroamphetamine. However, it is not likely to be different in its treatment recommendations or side effects profile. Its extended-release formulation (Adderall XR), using the extended-bead technology (50% IR and 50% delayed-release), has a longer and probably more effective duration of action, generally considered to be 10 to 12 hours in duration. It can also be sprinkled on food for those who have difficulty swallowing capsules.

Spencer and colleagues assessed the efficacy and safety of extended-release mixed amphetamine salts 10, 20, 30, and 40 mg/day in a 4-week, randomized, double-blind, placebo-controlled study in 287 adolescents aged 13 to 17 years.[24] Adolescents treated with all four doses of extended-release mixed amphetamine salts exhibited statistically significant ($P < 0.001$) improvement in mean ADHD-IV rating scale total scores compared with placebo at all weeks throughout the 4-week study. On the CGI-I scale at endpoint, compared with placebo, a higher percentage of patients in all active-treatment groups were considered improved (**Figure 5.11**). Adverse events, predominantly mild to moderate in intensity, were more frequent with extended-release mixed amphetamine salts than with placebo and included anorexia/decreased appetite, headache, insomnia, abdominal pain, and weight loss.

Lisdexamfetamine

Lisdexamfetamine (Vyvanse) is a prodrug that converts to dextroamphetamine in the blood stream due to the action of a peptidase that cleaves the lysine molecule. As a prodrug, it does not become active as dextroamphet-

FIGURE 5.11 — Percentage of Patients Improved vs Not Improved at Study Endpoint: Mixed Amphetamine Salts Extended-Release vs Placebo

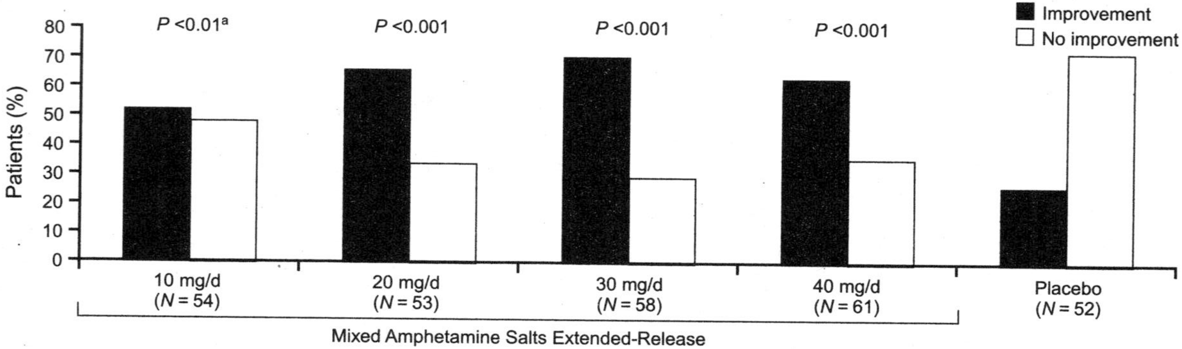

Improvement included CGI-I categories "very much improved" and "much improved"; no improvement included all other CGI-I categories.

[a] P value was based on the general association Cochran-Mantel-Haenszel statistic with adjustment for pooled center comparing the treatment groups. A closed testing procedure was used to test for a difference between each active treatment group and the placebo group, beginning with 40 mg vs placebo and stopping when significance ($P<0.05$) was not reached.

Adapted from: Spencer TJ, et al. *Clin Ther*. 2006;28:266-279.

amine until after it is metabolized. This characteristic lowers the ability for it to be diverted and abused via intranasal or intravenous routes. However, because it is metabolized into dextroamphetamine, it has similar restrictions as a prescription (class II) as other stimulant medications. The conversion of lisdexamfetamine to dextroamphetamine is not affected by GI pH and is unlikely to be affected by alterations in normal GI transit times. The pharmacokinetic profile of lisdexamfetamine is consistent with its prodrug chemical structure and is not dependent on type of formulation. Lisdexamfetamine capsules can be dissolved in water for patients who have difficulty swallowing. The metabolic process also results in a predictable time to peak plasma levels of dextroamphetamine and longer duration of action, usually only requiring once-a-day administration to provide 12-hour coverage.

Lisdexamfetamine is approved for the treatment of ADHD in adults and in children 6 to 12 years of age. One randomized, double-blind, crossover study in children aged 6 to 12 years with ADHD compared the efficacy of lisdexamfetamine with placebo and mixed amphetamine salts in a laboratory classroom setting.[25] The primary outcome measure was the SKAMP rating subscales (attention and deportment). Response to stimulant medications was assessed by the Permanent Product Measure of Performance (PERMP), a validated 10-minute written math test. Lisdexamfetamine treatment significantly improved SKAMP scores for deportment and attention (**Figure 5.12**, *top*) as well as PERMP-attempted and PERMP-correct scores (**Figure 5.12**, *bottom*).

Another randomized, double-blind, placebo-controlled study was performed in 420 adults aged 18 to 55 years with moderate to severe ADHD (*DSM-IV-TR* criteria).[26] Following a 7- to 28-day washout, patients were randomized to receive 30, 50, or 70 mg/day lisdexamfetamine or placebo, respectively, for 4 weeks (N=119, 117, 122, and 62, respectively). The 50- and 70-mg/day groups underwent forced-dose titration. The primary efficacy measure was the clinician-determined ADHD Rating Scale (ADHD-RS). At study endpoint, improvements in ADHD-RS scores in all three active

FIGURE 5.12 — Time-Course Changes in SKAMP and PERMP Scores Across Assessment Day in School-Age Children in a Laboratory Classroom Setting: Lisdexamfetamine Dimesylate, Mixed Amphetamine Salts Extended-Release, and Placebo

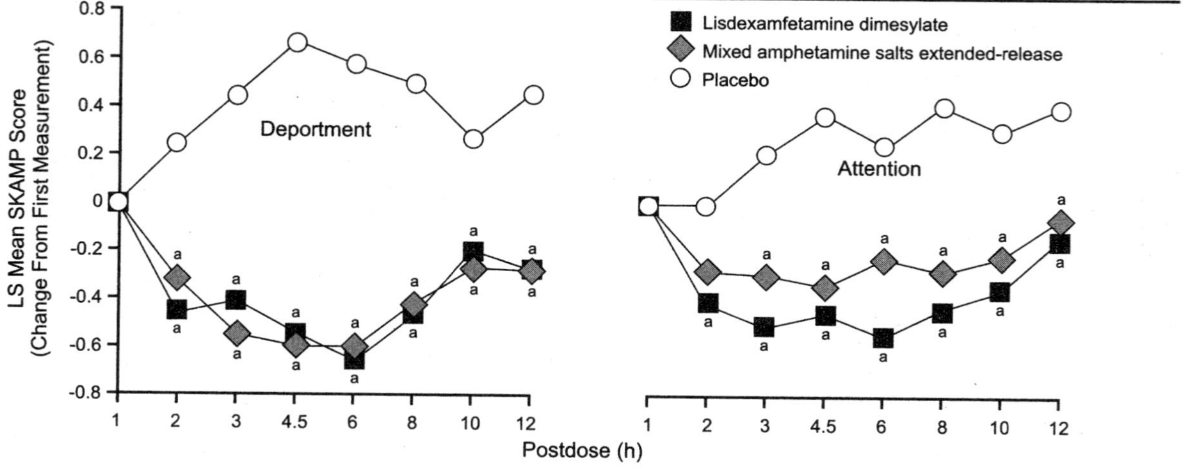

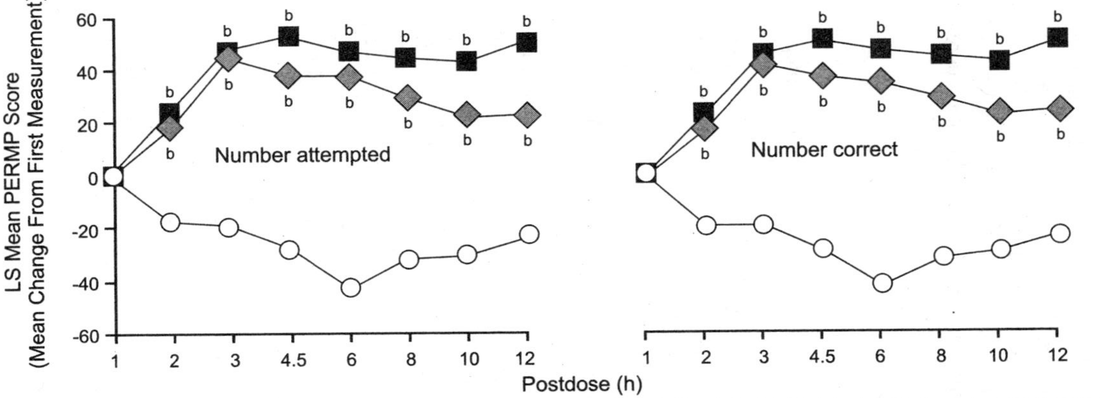

[a] $P<0.05$ vs placebo; $N=50$.
[b] $P<0.001$ vs placebo; $N=50$.

Adapted from: Biederman J, et al. *Biol Psychiatry*. 2007;62:970-976.

treatment groups were significantly (P <0.0001) greater for each lisdexamfetamine dose relative to placebo, with no differences between doses. In addition, there were significant differences compared with placebo in each lisdexamfetamine group beginning at week 1 and for each week throughout the study (**Figure 5.13**). Lisdexamfetamine was well tolerated. Adverse events were generally mild and included dry mouth, decreased appetite, and insomnia.

■ Nonstimulant Medications

Atomoxetine

Atomoxetine (Strattera) is a selective norepinephrine reuptake inhibitor. Its efficacy in treating patients with ADHD is based on >30 randomized control studies and it is approved by the FDA for treating ADHD in children, adolescents, and adults. Wilens and associates performed a meta-analysis of long-term efficacy from 13 trials of atomoxetine (six double-blind, seven open-label) in 601 adolescents (12 to 18 years of age) with ADHD.[27] ADHD Rating Scale IV scores showed significant (P <0.001) improvement from baseline over the first 3 months and remained significantly improved up to 24 months without dosage escalation (**Figure 5.14**).

Atomoxetine has a half-life of 4 to 19 hours and is typically prescribed once per day but can also be given in two divided doses. The common side effects of atomoxetine include appetite suppression, GI upset, and somnolence. Rarely, hepatotoxicity can occur and reports of increased suicidal ideation have prompted the FDA to issue a warning to monitor for this issue.

Atomoxetine is metabolized through the cytochrome P-450 2D6 pathway. There are some patients who are slow metabolizers, while most are extensive metabolizers. The clinical relevance of identifying slower metabolizers is not yet clear. Atomoxetine does not have abuse potential and is therefore is not a class II medication, which allows for it to be refilled and called in over the telephone. It does not provide the rapid behavioral changes seen with stimulant medication so that the improvements may not be as noticeable, particularly to patients and families who have utilized stimulant medi-

FIGURE 5.13 — Change From Baseline in ADHD-RS Total Scores at Each Week in Patients Taking Lisdexamfetamine vs Placebo: ITT Population

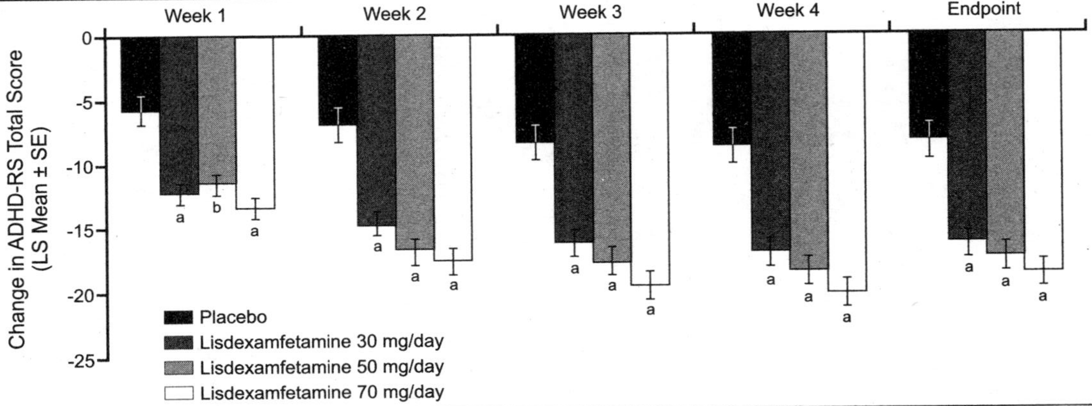

[a] P <0.0001 vs placebo.
[b] P <0.001 vs placebo.

Adler LA, et al. *J Clin Psychiatry*. 2008;69:1364-1373.

FIGURE 5.14 — Mean ADHD-RS-IV Total Scores for Adolescents Over 2 Years' Treatment With Atomoxetine

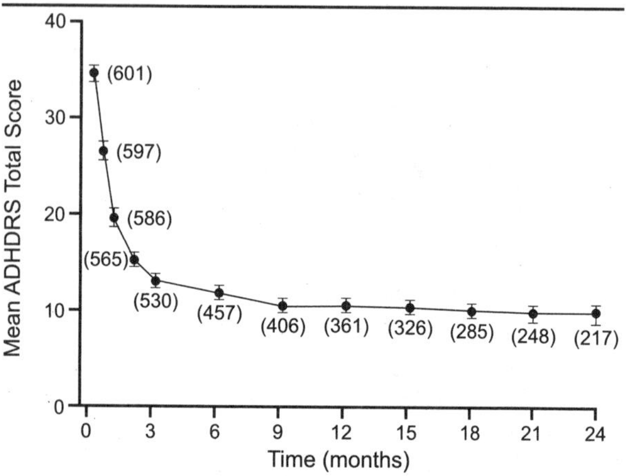

Wilens TE, et al. *J Pediatr*. 2006;149:112-119.

cations prior to a trial with atomoxetine. The full effects of a particular dose often take several weeks to become apparent and therefore dose titrations need to occur more slowly than with the stimulant medications. The slower changes emphasize the importance of monitoring the core symptoms through interviews and rating scales to assess the effect of the medication during titration since the changes are likely to be more subtle. While the effects documented in the controlled trials were for the daytime period, there is a suggestion that the medication effects may last >10 hours.

Non–FDA-Approved Medications That Have Been Used to Treat ADHD

The medications in this section have not been approved by the FDA for use in individuals with ADHD. These medications have not had sufficient evidence to demonstrate their efficacy, have more severe side effects, or have a narrower margin of safety. They are not recommended for use unless the stimulant medications and atomoxetine have been tried first and proved to be ineffective or have resulted in significant side effects. Behavioral interventions with better efficacy evidence should also be tried as well in these situations before trying the nonapproved medications.

■ Tricyclic Antidepressants

The tricyclic antidepressants used to treat patients with ADHD have generally been imipramine (Tofranil), desipramine (Norpramin), and nortriptyline (Pamelor). Their mechanism of action is to inhibit the reuptake of serotonin and norepinephrine, but they also have anticholinergic effects. Their efficacy in the treatment of ADHD has been supported by approximately 20 randomized-controlled trial studies. The tricyclic antidepressant medications are long-acting and take several days to achieve a therapeutic level. Their mean half-life is 28 to 36 hours and the average daily dose is 25 to 150 mg (1-5 mg/kg).

The minor side effects of the tricyclic antidepressant medications include sedation, anticholinergic effects, and anorexia, but the most significant side effect is arrhythmia. Most of the arrhythmias have been related to overdoses because of the narrow margin of safety, but at least for desipramine, there is a report of a sudden death at a therapeutic level. When prescribing the tricyclic antidepressant medications, it is important to monitor ECGs at baseline and then at each major dose change until an optimal dose is achieved. Blood levels should also be monitored to maintain a level between 150-250 ng/mL.

■ Alpha-Adrenergic Medications

The alpha-adrenergic medications used to treat patients with ADHD are clonidine (Catapres) and guanfacine (Tenex). While they were approved as antihypertensive agents, they are also alpha-noradrenergic agonists that affect the CNS. However, their evidence of efficacy in treating patients with ADHD is limited to two studies. More recently, additional studies completed on a long-acting form of guanfacine are under consideration by the FDA for approval. The alpha-adrenergic medications are slower in action than stimulants, with a half-life of 24 to 36 hours. The average daily dose is 0.5/5 and 4/40 mg/day for clonidine/guanfacine, respectively.

The side effects of the alpha-adrenergic medications include sedation, fatigue, anorexia, dry mouth, and hypotension. There have been several cases of sudden death in patients treated with a combination of clonidine and methylphenidate, but it could not be confirmed that the deaths were due to the medications. It is also important to taper the medication slowly when discontinuing its use and to monitor the patient's blood pressure closely while the patient is on the medication. A common use of clonidine is as an aid to sleep, a common problem in individuals with ADHD.

■ Bupropion

Bupropion (Wellbutrin) is an antidepressive medication whose mechanism of action is mostly unclear. It is a weak dopamine agonist, and it decreases whole-body norepinephrine levels, but neither of these effects appears to explain its clinical results. Its efficacy in treating patients with ADHD is derived from one multisite study in which it proved to be significantly better than placebo, but it was not as efficacious as stimulant medications. Bupropion has a half-life of 8 to 24 hours and is prescribed one, two, or three times per day, depending upon the formulation used. The side effects of bupropion include agitation, reduction in the seizure threshold, anorexia, insomnia, and nausea/vomiting. The appropriate dose range for treating children with bupropion is 1.4 mg to 6 mg/kg/day in divided doses, while adolescents and adults are usually treated with 150 mg to 300 mg/day. Bupropion is commonly used in those with comorbid ADHD and anxiety or depression in conjunction with stimulant medications.

■ Modafinil

Modafinil (Provigil) is a wakefulness-promoting agent approved to treat sleep disorders such as narcolepsy in adults. Three recent studies of modafinil have been completed in children with ADHD in a total of 638 patients and showed significant improvement compared with placebo. However, it was not approved by the FDA for the treatment of ADHD due to the development of Stevens-Johnson syndrome in two of the study patients. The half-life for modafinil is 15 hours in adults. The doses tested in the three controlled studies in children with ADHD were 340 mg for children <30 kg and 425 mg for those ≥30 kg in two of the studies. The third study used a variable titrated dose and had a mean dose of 361 mg. The dose was titrated at dose intervals of 85-mg increments at days 1, 3, 8, 15, and 22. The most common side effects were insomnia, headache, and decreased appetite.

Medication Management

5

Since the response to a particular medication is highly idiosyncratic, it is important to employ a systematic process to determine the most efficacious medication and dose for a patient. **Figure 5.15** is a medication algorithm for preschool-age patients; **Figure 5.16**, for primary school-age through adult patients. Since methylphenidate and amphetamines have similar properties, it is the personal preference of the patient, their family, and the clinician as to which medication to use initially. It is best to start at the lowest dose, the equivalent of 2.5 mg of methylphenidate for preschool-age children and 5 mg for children and adults, or 2.5 of an amphetamine compound for children and adults two or three times a day. The doses can be increased every 3 to 7 days at 2.5 or 5 mg/dose up to a maximum of 60 mg/day of methylphenidate (72 mg Concerta or 30 mg Daytrana) or 40 mg amphetamine (70 mg lisdexamfetamine). Based on clinical experience, some children and more adolescents and adults may require doses over the recommended maximums. Therefore, if a patient shows no side effects of a medication at the maximum dose but requires increased ADHD-symptom control, a careful upward titration of dose may be indicated. If, after reaching the highest dose of the first-choice stimulant medication group (methylphenidate or amphetamine), the patient is not manifesting improvement or significant side effects occur, it is worthwhile to try a medication from the other stimulant medication group.

The best method to determine a patient's initial response to the medication is to monitor the 18-core symptoms used to establish the diagnosis. Rating scales

FIGURE 5.15 — Medication Algorithm for Preschool-Age Patients

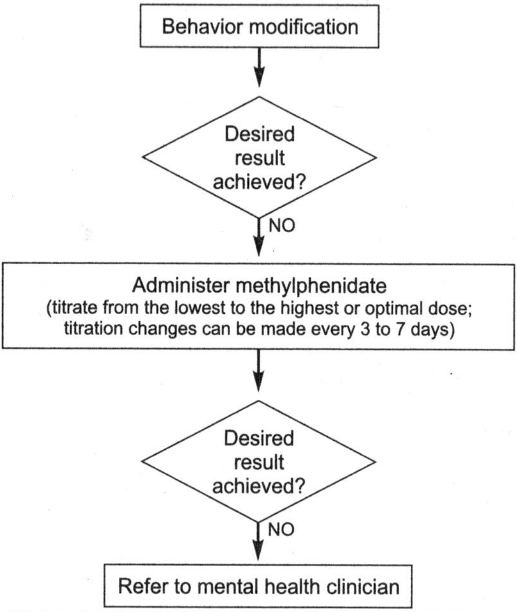

that are based on *DSM-IV* criteria, such as the Vanderbilt Rating Scales, can provide that information from parents and teachers. The clinician should try to achieve at least a 25% to 35% decrease in symptoms, although with many patients it is possible to achieve a 50% to 70% reduction. It is best when, if at all possible, information about the core symptoms comes from more than one source. In children, the sources usually consist of the parent and teacher since children are not accurate reporters of their own behaviors. However, adolescents and adults are typically the only source to offer their self-assessments of efficacy and adverse effects.

During the titration phase, it is possible to conduct the monitoring through phone calls, faxes, emails, or web-based data systems. For more long-term monitoring, it is helpful to have monthly visits for the first 3 to 6 months. In addition to checking height, weight, and blood pressure, it is possible to explore both beneficial and side effects in more detail. It is also a good time to

FIGURE 5.16 — Medication Algorithm for Primary School-Age Through Adult Patients

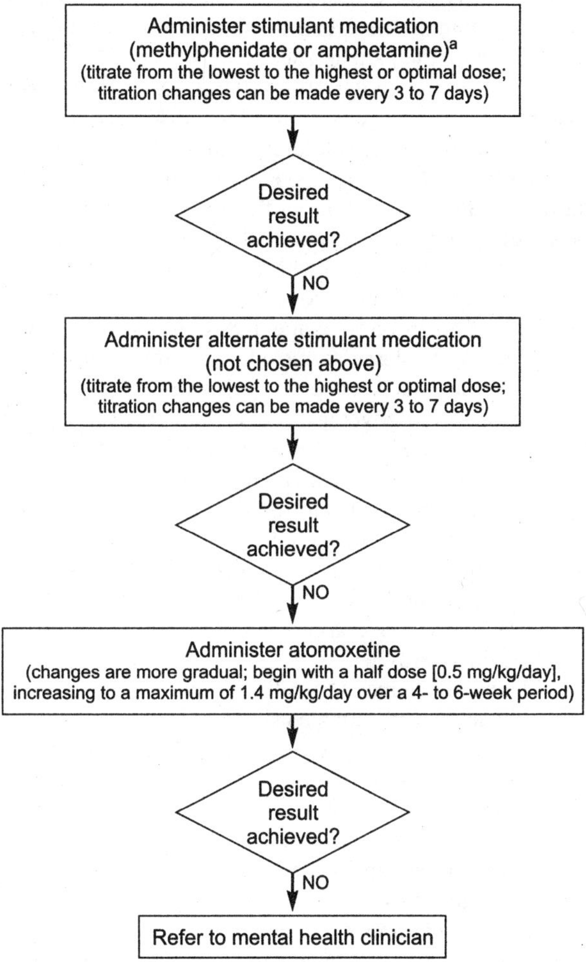

[a] Either of the two groups of stimulant medications can be offered initially, depending on the preference of the patient, their family, and the prescribing physician. Each group of stimulants is supplied in one of three categories: short-acting generic, long-acting brand names, and/or a dermal patch. After deciding which group is preferred, the clinician and patient need to select the category that is most acceptable, then titrate, beginning with the lowest dose.

review the target goals to determine if the changes in core symptoms are improving the function as defined by the goals. Subsequently, if the improvements remain stable, ongoing management can be spaced less frequently, depending on the patient's needs.

For stimulant medications, the length of time daily that requires coverage is an important discussion to have with the family. Those children with the inattentive type of condition who do not have much homework may be able to manage on 8 hours of coverage with weekend and summer holidays, particularly for families who desire to minimize the medication use as much as possible. Children with the combined type are more likely to need 12 hours of coverage and require medication 7 days a week. Adolescents and adults need to consider the times they are likely to be driving as important times to have medication coverage. College students may have more chaotic and varied days that become more difficult to arrange for broad coverage and may ask about using immediate-release formulations at targeted times, such as when studying, taking exams, or writing papers. Adolescents and young adults also have to be warned about preventing diversion of the medication and that if they are involved in that process, they can incur significant legal jeopardy.

Atomoxetine may be the first drug of choice for families who are uncomfortable using a controlled substance. There is also some suggestion that it may be of benefit for patients with comorbid anxiety or learning disabilities. While atomoxetine also requires some titration, it is different than for the stimulant medications because the effects are not as rapid. The changes are likely to occur more gradually over a 2- to 4-week period, although frequently some noticeable changes will occur after the first week. Since the changes may not be as noticeable, use of rating scales to monitor core symptoms can help to clarify the changes.

Many patients stop taking their medications after several years. While there are many patients who improve in their abilities to compensate for their core symptoms and can manage to function without medication, there are many who continue to see benefits on treatment. The extent to which a patient will continue to follow a treatment regimen is dependent on how much they know about their condition, how convenient it is to administer the treatment, how much benefit they perceive from the treatment, as well as the nature of any side effects. It is to this issue that the importance of treating ADHD as a chronic illness was discussed in the previous chapter.

REFERENCES

1. Bradley C. The behavior of children receiving benzedrine. *Am J Psychiatry.* 1937;94:577-585.
2. Swanson JM, Gupta S, Williams L, Agler D, Lerner M, Wigal S. Efficacy of a new pattern of delivery of methylphenidate for the treatment of ADHD: effects on activity level in the classroom and on the playground. *J Am Acad Child Adolesc Psychiatry.* 2002;41(11):1306-1314.
3. Spencer T, Biederman J, Wilens T, et al. A large, double-blind, randomized clinical trial of methylphenidate in the treatment of adults with attention-deficit/hyperactivity disorder. *Biol Psychiatry.* 2005;57(5):456-463.
4. Biederman J, Mick E, Surman C, et al. A randomized, placebo-controlled trial of OROS methylphenidate in adults with attention-deficit/hyperactivity disorder. *Biol Psychiatry.* 2006;59(9):829-835.
5. Greenhill L, Kollins S, Abikoff H, et al. Efficacy and safety of immediate-release methylphenidate treatment for preschoolers with ADHD. *J Am Acad Child Adolesc Psychiatry.* 2006;45(11):1284-1293.
6. Gleason MM, Egger HL, Emslie GJ, et al. Psychopharmacological treatment for very young children: contexts and guidelines. *J Am Acad Child Adolesc Psychiatry.* 2007;46(12):1532-1572.
7. Shaw P, Greenstein D, Lerch J, et al. Intellectual ability and cortical development in children and adolescents. *Nature.* 2006;440(7084):676-679.
8. Murphy K, Barkley RA. Attention deficit hyperactivity disorder in adults: comorbidities and adaptive impairments. *Compr Psychiatry.* 1996;37(6):393-401.
9. McGough JJ, Smalley SL, McCracken JT, et al. Psychiatric comorbidity in adult attention deficit hyperactivity disorder: findings from multiplex families. *Am J Psychiatry.* 2005;162(9):1621-1627.
10. Wigal T, Swanson JM, Regino R, et al. Stimulant medications for the treatment of ADHD: Efficacy and limitations. *Ment Retard Dev Disabil Res Rev.* 1999;5:215-224.

11. Ingram S, Hechtman L, Morgenstern G. Outcome issues in ADHD: adolescent and adult long-term outcome. *Ment Retard Dev Disabil Res Rev.* 1999;5:243-250.

12. Jensen PS, Arnold LE, Swanson JM, et al. 3-year follow-up of the NIMH MTA study. *J Am Acad Child Adolesc Psychiatry.* 2007;46(8):989-1002.

13. Efron D, Jarman F, Barker M. Methylphenidate versus dexamphetamine in children with attention deficit hyperactivity disorder: a double-blind, crossover trial. *Pediatrics.* 1997;100:1-7.

14. Greenhill LL, Findling RL, Swanson JM, et al. A double-blind, placebo-controlled study of modified-release methylphenidate in children with attention-deficit/ hyperactivity disorder. *Pediatrics.* 2002;109:E39.

15. Beiderman J, Quinn D, Weiss M, et al. Efficacy and safety of Ritalin LA, a new once-daily, extended-release dosage form of methylphenidate, in children with attention deficit hyperactivity disorder. *Pediatr Drugs.* 2003;5:833-841.

16. Wolraich ML, Greenhill LL, Pelham W, et al; on behalf of the Concerta Study Group. Randomized, controlled trial of OROS methylphenidate once a day in children with attention-deficit/ hyperactivity disorder. *Pediatrics.* 2001;108;883-892.

17. Muniz R, Brams M, Mao A, et al. Efficacy and safety of extended-release dexmethylphenidate compared with *d.l*-methylphenidate and placebo in the treatment of children with attention-deficit/ hyperactivity disorder: a 12-hour laboratory classroom study. *J Child Adolesc Psychopharmacol.* 2008;18:246-256.

18. McGough JJ, Wigal SB, Turnbow JM, et al. A randomized, double-blind, placebo-controlled laboratory classroom assessment of methylphenidate transdermal system in children with ADHD. *J Attent Disord.* 2006;9:476-485.

19. Tourette's Syndrome Study Group. Treatment of ADHD in children with tics: a randomized controlled trial. *Neurology.* 2002;58(4):527-536.

20. Avigan M. Review of AERS data from marketed safety experience during stimulant therapy: death, sudden death. Cardiovascular SAEs (including stroke): Department of Health and Human Services, Public Health Service, Food and Drug Administration, Center for Drug Evaluation and Research; April 27,2004, DO30403.

21. Vetter VL, Elia J, Erickson C, et al; American Heart Association Council on Cardiovascular Disease in the Young Congenital Cardiac Defects Committee. American Heart Association Council on Cardiovascular Nursing. Cardiovascular monitoring of children and adolescents with heart disease receiving stimulant drugs: a scientific statement from the American Heart Association Council

on Cardiovascular Disease in the Young Congenital Cardiac Defects Committee and the Council on Cardiovascular Nursing. *Circulation*. 2008;117(18):2407-2423.

22. Perrin JM, Friedman RA, Knilans, TK; the Black Box Working Group and Section on Cardiology and Cardiac Surgery. Cardiovascular Monitoring and Stimulant Drugs for Attention-Deficit/Hyperactivity Disorder. http://aappolicy.acppublications.org/cgi/reprint/pediatrics;122/2/451.pdf. Accessed March 30, 2009.

23. AAP/AHA Clarification Statement on Cardiovascular Evaluation and Monitoring of Children and adolescents with Heart Disease receiving Medication for ADHD http://americanheart.mediaroom.com/index.php?s=43&item=422. Accessed March 30, 2009.

24. Spencer TJ, Wilens TE, Biederman J, et al. Efficacy and safety of mixed amphetamine salts extended release (Adderall XR) in the management of attention-deficit/hyperactivity disorder in adolescent patients: a 4-week, randomized, double-blind, placebo-controlled, parallel-group study. *Clin Ther*. 2006;28:266-279.

25. Beiderman J, Boellner SW, Childress A, et al. Lisdexamfetamine dimesylate and mixed amphetamine salts extended release in children with ADHD: a double-blind, placebo-controlled, crossover analog classroom study. *Biol Psychiatry*. 2007;62:970-976.

26. Adler LA, Goodman DW, Kollins SH, et al, on behalf of the 303 Study Group. Double-blind, placebo-controlled study of the efficacy and safety of lisdexamfetamine dimesylate in adults with attention-deficit/hyperactivity disorder. *J Clin Psychiatry*. 2008;69:1364-1373.

27. Wilens TE, Newcorn JH, Kratochvil C, et al. Long-term atomoxetine treatment in adolescents with attention-deficit/hyperactivity disorder. *J Pediatr.* 2006;149:112-119.

6 Psychosocial Treatments

Psychosocial interventions include all of the interventions that employ counseling or behavior management. In children, the one most frequently employed and having the strongest scientific evidence for its efficacy is behavior-modification training for the significant caretakers (parents and teachers) in the child's environment.[1] Social skills therapy tries to address the deficits that many children with ADHD have in social situations, but because of the difficulty that children with ADHD have in generalizing what they learn, there is limited evidence for its efficacy unless the training takes place in actual situations with other children.[1] Family therapy may be helpful, particularly on issues such as sibling relationships, but the evidence for its efficacy is weaker. Play and cognitive therapies have not been found to be efficacious treatments for children with ADHD.[1] The number of studies on behavioral interventions in adults is very limited. The most common behavioral interventions for adults are cognitive behavioral therapy, organizational and educational tutoring, and ADHD coaching. While coaching utilizes a simple and cost-effective practical approach, it has yet to be studied under rigorous conditions.

Parent-Training Programs

The most common behavior modification intervention for children is parent training. This training may take different forms depending on the severity of the behavioral problems. With children whose behavioral problems are mild and with parents who are adept at behavior management, simple advice from their primary care clinician combined with reading material may suffice, although such interventions have not been rigorously studied. **Table 6.1** provides some books that can be recommended.

For parents who require more intense instruction, most communities offer group-training programs in

TABLE 6.1 — Books and Web Resources Recommended for Parent Training

Books

- Kazdin AE, Weisz, JR, eds. *Evidence-based Psychotherapies for Children and Adolescents*. New York: Guilford Press; 2003:224-240.
- Forehand R, Long N. *Parenting the Strong-Willed Child.* New York: McGraw-Hill; 2002.
- Phelan TW. *1-2-3 Magic: Effective Discipline for Children 2-12*. Glen Ellyn, IL: Parentmagic, Inc; 2004.

Web Resources[a]

- NYU Child Study Center (www.aboutourkids.org)
- Center for Effective Parenting (www.parenting-ed.org)
- Child and Family WebGuide (www.cfw.tufts.edu)
- National Parent Information Network (www.npin.org)
- Children and Adults with ADHD (CHADD) (www.chadd.org)

[a] Most taken from *Parenting the Strong-Willed Child* written by Forehand and Long.

Accessed March 30, 2009.

which parents receive instructions in behavior-modification techniques, role play the techniques, and then apply them to their children between classes. These programs usually meet weekly and last 8 to 14 weeks. The international support organization CHADD has developed such a program and combines it with information about ADHD to help families better understand the condition. **Table 6.2** presents some of the common programs available.

When parents find it difficult to understand or implement the behavioral techniques and/or their children demonstrate more severe behavior problems, individualized training tailored to the family's needs is required. The most severe situations, short of removing a child from the home, may require implementing the parent training directly in the home or utilizing a day-treatment situation that can train the parent while intensely shaping the child's behavior. An evidenced-based individual parent-training program is Parent-Child Interaction Therapy.[2] This program utilizes supervised skill training in working with both the parent and the child and utilizes an auditory transmitter to provide direct supervision while observing

TABLE 6.2 — Parenting Programs

Helping the Noncompliant Child[a]

- Child age: 3-8 years
- Format: Parent and child seen together in weekly individual sessions
- Length of treatment: 10 sessions (60-90 minutes each)
- Setting: clinic or home
- Key features: Parents are taught to change negative parent-child interactions by giving positive attention for appropriate behaviors, ignoring minor misbehaviors, giving clear directions, and following through with appropriate consequences for compliance and non-compliance. Intended as a secondary prevention program. Involves modeling, role-playing, and in vivo training, and continues until each skill is mastered.

Incredible Years (IY)[b]

- IY Parent training program:
  - Child age: 2-10 years
  - Format: group therapy (8-12 parents per group)
  - Length of treatment: 13 sessions (2 hours each)
  - Setting: clinic or school
  - Key features: Uses videotape modeling to teach parents skills for increasing children's positive behaviors and applying effective discipline skills with their child. Also teaches parents to help their child learn problem-solving skills.
- IY Child Training:
  - Child age: 3-8 years
  - Format: group therapy with six children per group
  - Length of treatment: 22 weeks (2 hours each week)
  - Setting: clinic or school
  - Key features: Uses video vignettes to facilitate discussion of problem-solving and social skills. Typically completed in conjunction with the IY parent training program, although evidence suggests it is effective in improving children's behavior alone.

Parent-Child Interaction Therapy (PCIT)[c]

- Child age: 3-6 years
- Format: individual sessions with parent and child seen together
- Length of treatment: 12-16 sessions (one hour each)
- Setting: clinic

Continued

- Key features: Teaches parents to use play-therapy skills to enhance the parent-child interaction by giving positive attention to children when they are behaving appropriately and ignoring minor misbehavior. Also instructs parents in how to give effective direction to children and implement effective discipline strategies. Once parents have been taught the skills by the therapist, further sessions involve the therapist coaching the parent using a bug-in-the-ear device as they use the skills with their child, providing immediate feedback to parents and guiding them in their use of the skills.

Parent Management Training Oregon Model (PMTO)[d]

- Child age: 3-12 years
- Format: individual sessions with parent and child seen together
- Length of treatment: varies (10-17 sessions reported on average)
- Setting: clinic
- Key features: PMTO teaches parents basic behavioral principles for modifying child behavior, encourages parents to monitor child behaviors, and assists parents in developing and implementing behavior-modification programs to improve targeted child-behavior problems.

Positive Parenting Program (Triple P)[e]

- Triple P Standard Individual Treatment:
  - Child age: 3-4 years
  - Format: group, individual, or self-directed
  - Length of treatment: 12 sessions
  - Setting: clinic
  - Key features: Triple P is a multilevel system of treatment, with 5 levels of intensity designed to match child and family needs based on problem severity. Levels 1 through 3 are prevention programs. Standard Triple P is a parent-training program for disruptive behavior delivered by mental health providers. Parents are taught 17 core parenting skills (eg, talking with children, physical affection, attention, setting limits, planned ignoring) designed to increase positive child behaviors and decrease negative child behaviors.
- Triple P Enhanced Treatment:
  - Child age: 3-4 years
  - Format: individual
  - Length of treatment: 11 sessions (60-90 minutes each)
  - Setting: clinic

Continued

– Key features: The Triple P Enhanced Treatment is designed for families with child behavior problems and family dysfunction. Program modules include teaching parents skills stressed in the standard treatment program, home visits to enhance parenting skills, partner support skills, and mood management/stress coping skills.

[a] Forehand R, McMahon R. *Helping the Noncompliant Child: A Clinician's Guide to Parent Training*. New York: Guilford; 1981.

[b] Webster-Stratton C, Reid M. The incredible years parents, teachers, and children training series: a multifaceted treatment approach for young children with conduct problems. In: Kazdin A, Weisz JR, eds. *Evidence-based Psychotherapies for Children and Adolescents*. New York: Guilford Press; 2004:224-240.

[c] Brinkmeyer M, Eyberg SM. Parent-child interaction therapy for oppositional children. In: Kazdin A, Weisz JR, eds. *Evidence-based Psychotherapies for Children and Adolescents*. New York: Guilford Press; 2004:204-223.

[d] Patterson G, et al. *A Social Learning Approach to Family Intervention: Families With Aggressive Children (Vol 1)*. Eugene, OR: Castalia; 1975.

[e] Sanders M. Triple P-positive parenting program: towards an empirically validated multilevel parenting and family support strategy for the prevention of behavior and emotional problems in children. *Clin Child Fam Psychol Rev*. 1999;2:71-90.

6

the parent applying the techniques directly with their own child. This more intense coaching process has been demonstrated to be efficacious for most parents.[3]

Whether a group or individual approach is utilized, parent training usually consists of the five elements presented in **Table 6.3**.

It is essential for parents to provide positive attention and reinforcement to their children. Many times, because of their child's difficult behaviors, parents of children with ADHD get into a cycle in which most of their interactions are negative and involve punishment for negative behaviors. Unless they are able to develop a systematic method for providing quality time in the form of positive attention and reinforcing the children for appropriate behaviors, the punishments will be less effective and the desired goals will not be achieved. Positive attention requires providing undivided attention to the child during activities. The parents also need to learn to recognize and reward appropriate behaviors. They need to provide immediate rewards that may be no more than praising

TABLE 6.3 — Principal Elements of Parent Training

- Providing children with clear commands and rules and keeping them aware of those rules
- Providing children with positive attention and reinforcement for positive behaviors
- Providing punishment and the removal of the positive attention for rule violations and inappropriate behaviors
- Providing rewards, and punishments that are contingent and timely
- Providing consistent rules, rewards, and punishments

their children immediately after the child completes an appropriate behavior. In addition, for more meaningful longer-term achievements, the parents need to develop rewards that are attractive to their children. These rewards may entail additional privileges or tangible rewards, requiring several instances of appropriate behaviors before they are earned.

A commonly used systematic method of providing reinforcement is a token system. A token system consists of identifying the appropriate behaviors parents want to increase in their child. The three or four most appropriate behaviors are targeted, and the child can earn points for performing the appropriate behavior. As an example, if the parent wants their child to say please when the child requests something, the child can earn points every time they use please appropriately. For young children between 3 and 6 or 7 years of age, tangible tokens may work better than points. The parents need to set up a system, such as a chart, to keep track of the points, and the child needs to know how many points are needed to achieve a reward. The target behaviors and the number of points required to earn rewards can be revised as the child progresses or if the system does not seem to be working. The rewards can be special privileges (eg, increased television time or increased time with a parent) or they can be tangible (eg, baseball cards). Immediate praise for earning points can help to enhance the effects. In the adolescent and older school-age child, they need to be part of the negotiations to define the rules, rewards for accomplishments, and punishments for infractions. It is frequently helpful to formalize this process and develop a written contract that is signed by both the parent and the child.

A positive system alone is usually not sufficient to control the behavior of a child with ADHD. Some punishment system is also required for rule violations and inappropriate behaviors. Effective forms of punishment are time-outs for younger children and removal of privileges for older children and adolescents. With a token system, a cost response can also be employed. In that system, points are removed for rule violations and inappropriate behaviors. The child requires clear messages about the rules and what are inappropriate behaviors.

School Services

Children with ADHD can receive services from their schools based on the Rehabilitation Act (504)[4] for milder cases and the Individuals with Disability Education Act (IDEA) for more severe cases. The Rehabilitation Act (504) requires schools to provide accommodations so that the child can function in their class. Almost all children with the diagnosis of ADHD are eligible. However, the act does not provide any added compensation to the school. Therefore, the adaptations provided are often limited in nature and the procedures may vary greatly from school to school. The adaptations include preferential class seating, assignment and homework reduction or modification, test modifications (eg, extended time), or taking tests in a less-distracting setting. In some schools, a school psychologist is available to help the teacher set up a behavioral program.

The IDEA is a much more comprehensive program, but is only available to those children with ADHD when the ADHD significantly interferes with their ability to learn, children whose other comorbid condition results in more impaired behavior, or children with cognitive comorbidities, such as learning disabilities or significant sensory or motor impairments. The school system is required to provide comprehensive testing that includes intellectual and achievement testing, as well as speech and language assessments, and additional testing if appropriate. Testing provided by an external source, such as a private psychologist, can be used in place of the school testing if the school personnel feel it is accurate, but most frequently that testing has to be obtained at the parents' expense, whereas public schools can provide testing conducted by their personnel or contractors at no charge to the family.

If a child qualifies for services (for ADHD it falls under the category of "Other Health Impaired"), the school system must develop an individual education plan (IEP) with clearly measurable goals. The services must be provided so that the child is placed as close to the mainstream as possible (least-restricted environment). For most children with ADHD, the accommodations will consist of a small portion of the day spent in the resource room with a teacher trained in special education or with help from an aid in the classroom. Speech and language and occupational therapy services are also provided if necessary for language or motor impairments. The whole process from obtaining the testing through providing the services must be accomplished with informed parental consent. The IDEA has been able to implement specific national guidelines and services because the schools are provided increased revenues based on the number of students they serve who qualify for special education and the severity of the students' needs. The testing and parent conferences need to be sensitive to different cultures, languages, and disabilities of the students and their families.

The clinician's role is to inform the parents about the services that are available at school and the procedures required to access the services. Informational materials are usually available for families through the state departments of education. In most situations, it is helpful for the parent to send a letter to the school principal requesting that an educational evaluation be performed. The school district or state departments of education frequently produce pamphlets that explain the services and procedures, and it is helpful to have that information available in the clinician's office for families when a diagnosis of ADHD is made.

As noted previously, social skills are a common deficit in children with ADHD. Social-skills training may be helpful, but only if it is provided in social situations (eg, classroom or other group activities) so that the training can be applied in the real context with the opportunity for practice and feedback.

Communication Between Parents, Schools, and Clinicians

The daily report card (DRC) is a useful tool to coordinate behavior management between teachers and parents and to provide the clinician with useful information by which they can measure the effects of medication on the performance of the child in the classroom. It provides a good means of communication between parents and teachers, is inexpensive, and requires minimal effort on the teacher's part, yet provides documented benefits for the children. The teacher, parent, and child together define four to five activities that have been problematic for the child. An example is provided in **Table 6.4**. To be successful, the DRC needs to target individualized behaviors, establish procedures for monitoring, give feedback to the child for the behaviors, provide feedback to the parents for the behaviors, and provide a reward for positive consequences. Generally, a 20% improvement over baseline is targeted for each goal, and the child should have a success rate of 66%. If the success rate is lower, it will not provide enough encouragement, and if it is close to 100%, the tasks are too easily accomplished. As the child improves, the requirements for success should be modified to maintain the same level of success. Positive reports should be rewarded with reinforcements that are of value to the child, such as increased privileges or tangible prizes. For adolescents, communication with teachers can be more difficult. It is often necessary for parents or caregivers to expend energy to obtain regular feedback on assignments, behaviors, and test results.

Adolescent and Adult Behavioral Interventions

Counseling and coaching are adjunctive modalities of therapy that can play a critical role for adolescents and adults with ADHD. Many individuals benefit from

TABLE 6.4 — Daily Report Card

Child's Name ______________________________ Date __________

	Special	Language Arts	Math	Reading	Social Studies/ Science
Follows class rules with no more than 3 rule violations per period	Y N	Y N	Y N	Y N	Y N
Completes class assignments within the designated time	Y N	Y N	Y N	Y N	Y N
Completes class assignments at 80% accuracy	Y N	Y N	Y N	Y N	Y N
Complies with teacher requests (no more than 3 instances of noncompliance per period)	Y N	Y N	Y N	Y N	Y N
No more than 3 instances of calling out per period	Y N	Y N	Y N	Y N	Y N

Other

Follows attendance rules	Y N					
Follows recess rules	Y N					
Total Numbers of Yeses	______					
Teacher's Initials		____	____	____	____	____

Comments: ______________________________

____

____

counseling with a focus on the individual, on relationships, substance abuse disorder (SUD), educational and/or employment achievement, or organizational strategies. Therapists with experience with patients with ADHD can be an invaluable asset in the development of a coordinated management strategy. Recently, many adolescents and adults with ADHD have benefited from coaching as a way to help them maintain focus on daily activities and to set priorities. Coaching can be accomplished in person or by email or telephone, and is being used with increasing frequency as a lower-cost alternative to help individuals with ADHD stay on task and accomplish their goals. Finally, academic or employment accommodations, as provided for in the Americans with Disabilities Act, should be pursued to help individuals with ADHD succeed to the level of their abilities. Adults should also be educated about the accommodations that they can receive at their places of employment or education under the same act. A variety of Internet-based resources are available including on-line support (see http://groups.yahoo.com/search?query=ADHD. Accessed March 30, 2009).

In summary, there are evidenced-based behavioral interventions and school accommodations that are important to consider as part of the management plan that clinicians develop for their patients with ADHD. These should be a part of the management plan for the majority of patients of all ages with ADHD.

REFERENCES

1. Pelham WE Jr, Wheeler T, Chronis A. Empirically supported psychosocial treatments for attention deficit hyperactivity disorder. *J Clin Child Psychol.* 1998;27:190-205.

2. Herschell AD, Calzada EJ, Eyberg SM, McNeil CB. Parent-child interaction therapy: new directions in research. *Cogn Behav Pract.* 2002;9:9-16.

3. Eisenstadt TH, Eyberg SM, McNeil CB, Newcomb K, Funderburk B. Parent-child interaction therapy with behavior problem children: relative effectiveness of two stages and overall treatment outcome. *J Clin Psychol.* 1993;22:42-51.

4. Davila RR, Williams ML, MacDonald JT. Memorandum on clarification of policy to address the needs of children with attention deficit disorders within general and/or special education. In: Parker HC, ed. *The ADD Hyperactivity Handbook for Schools.* Plantation, FL: Impact Publications Inc; 1992:261-268.

7 Alternative Treatments

So far we have presented those treatments that have reasonable evidence for their efficacy and safety. A number of treatments besides stimulant medications and behavioral interventions have been promoted for patients with ADHD, but there is not yet sufficient evidence for their efficacy and safety. These can be categorized into the broad groups of diets, dietary supplements, alternative medications, exercises, and biofeedback.

Diets

For many years, diets have been prominent in the interventions recommended for children with ADHD. The three diets commonly suggested to treat children with ADHD have been the:

- Feingold diet
- Oligoantigenic (oligoallergenic) or Few-Foods diet
- Restricted sugar diet.

■ Feingold Diet

The Feingold diet was proposed by an allergist, Dr. Ben Feingold, who suggested that some children with ADHD had an allergic-type reaction to certain dietary elements.[1] These elements included additives, preservatives, food dyes, and salicylate compounds. His clinical impression was that a number of children with hyperactivity improved when placed on a diet devoid of these elements. However, subsequent blinded studies found very few children responded adversely when challenged with dyes or additives (approximately 1% of the children studied).[2] Blinded studies consisted of challenging children with an offending element or placebo after the children were placed on the restricted diet or comparing periods of time when the children were on the restricted diet to periods on a placebo diet. The studies were not consistent about which dyes and preservatives were tested. Maintaining the diet, if strictly adhered to, can provide inadequate vitamin C, although current recommendations have dropped the natural salicylate restrictions so that the low amount of vitamin C should no longer be a problem. In addition, the diet requires significant time for food preparation, and parent-child conflicts often increase over compliance. The implementation of the Feingold diet has decreased, but the principle of eliminating additives and preservatives has been incorporated into the Few-Foods Diet discussed next. There has also been a recent study in normal children whose behavior was worsened when challenged with dyes and preservatives, but it is not clear how these results relate to children with ADHD.[3]

■ Oligoantigenic (Oligoallergenic) or Few-Foods Diet

Similar to the Feingold diet, the oligoantigenic (oligoallergenic) or Few-Foods diet hypothesizes that some children with ADHD are responding adversely to specific foods and dietary ingredients.[4] As with the Feingold diet, this diet restricts additives, dyes, and preservatives, but it also initially limits the patient's diet to two meats, two vegetables, two fruits, and two carbohydrates. If a positive response is seen after several weeks, other foods are gradually reintroduced, one at a time, to determine which foods adversely affect the patient's behavior. The hypothesis is that affected individuals have a sensitivity to certain foods that adversely affects their behavior. Approximately five studies have examined this intervention with blinding and controlled conditions.[5] While some effects were demonstrated, the methodologic weaknesses, such as problems with blinding, preclude making a definitive conclusion about the efficacy of the diet. The diet requires significant time for food preparation, and parent-child conflicts often increase over compliance.

■ Sugar-Restriction Diet

Sugar was first believed to adversely affect behavior based on several studies finding an association between worsening behavior and increased sugar intake.[6] Those recommending the elimination of sugar to control behaviors have usually referred to refined and added sugars as the offending agents. These sugars are usually sucrose or fructose. In a total of 23 rigorous studies that have been completed, no association between sugar and behavior was found.[6] The main side effect of the diet is that it is difficult to make children comply, and pursuing compliance usually increases parent-child conflicts. It also requires a good deal of food preparation to maintain the diet.

Dietary Supplements

The dietary supplements recommended for treating children with ADHD include essential fatty acids (EFAs), megavitamins, zinc, antioxidants, and herbs.[7]

7

■ Essential Fatty Acids

EFAs, such as omega-3 fatty acids, are a family of long-chain polyunsaturated fatty acids essential to brain development and neuronal functioning. Therefore, there has been some interest in the possibility that a deficiency of them may adversely affect behavior. The two primary EFAs under consideration are linoleic and linolenic acids. There have been several observational studies that have found lower levels of omega-3 fatty acids in persons with ADHD.[8,9] However, the results from randomized control trials of enhanced dietary intake of the fatty acids are somewhat unconvincing. Two studies found no improvement in ADHD-related behaviors[10,11] and one study showed improvement in three of its 14 measures.[12] There are no known physical risks associated with omega-3 fatty acid treatment at this time.

■ Megavitamins

Megavitamins consist of large quantities (at least 10 times the recommended daily allowance) of most vitamins. The assumption is that there is a need for a highly complex biochemical balance for optimal mental functioning. There is no clear evidence for their efficacy, and there is the potential physical side effect of elevated liver function test results.[13,14]

■ **Zinc**

Zinc has been recommended for the treatment of some patients with ADHD on the basis of finding some children with zinc deficiency based on hair analysis. Treatment with zinc has not been studied vigorously, and no physical risks have yet been identified.[15] The only potential problem is maintaining compliance and the parent-child conflict it causes, although they are less problematic than maintaining a total diet as described previously.

■ **Antioxidants**

Antioxidants are believed to have immunologic and neuroprotective effects. Antioxidants that have been promoted for use in ADHD are melatonin, ginkgo biloba, and pycnogenol. There have been no scientific studies of their effects on patients with ADHD, and their potential side effects are unknown.[15]

■ **Herbal Compounds**

Herbal compounds have mainly been recommended for treating patients with ADHD because of their sedative properties. The herbal compounds recommended are chamomile, kava hops, lemon balm, valerian root, and passionflower. There have not been any rigorous studies of their efficacy in patients with ADHD, and their potential side effects remain unknown.[15]

Alternative Medications

■ **Antifungal Agents**

The hypothesis behind antifungal therapy is that children treated on multiple occasions with broad-spectrum antibiotics, such as for otitis media, have alterations in their intestinal flora making them susceptible to the growth of *Candida* and the absorption of *Candida* toxins. These toxins may then produce behavioral disturbances. The treatment consists of using antifungal agents, such as nystatin or ketoconazole, and eliminating sugar and foods made with molds and yeast from the diet. The treatment has not been tested in a rigorous manner and, as with other dietary interventions, the parent needs to devote a good deal of time to the treatment and food preparations, and there can be conflicts between parent and child over compliance.[15] In addition, there are the potential side effects of the antifungal agents.

■ Nootropic Medications

Nootropic medications are cerebral metabolic enhancers that stave off aging. Those recommended for individuals with ADHD are piracetam and dimethylaminoethanol. There have been no rigorous studies of their efficacy, and there are no reported significant side effects, although the side effects have also not been studied systematically in children.[15]

Exercises and Training

7

In addition to dietary and medicinal interventions, there have been a group of therapies proposed that involve exercises or training, including:

- EEG biofeedback
- Sensory integration training
- Auditory training.[16]

■ EEG Biofeedback

EEG biofeedback works on the premise that the EEG pattern reflects an individual's behavior, and that if one can change their EEG pattern with suppression of theta-wave activity and enhancement of beta-wave production, their behavior will change. Furthermore, it is hypothesized that individuals can be trained to control these activities.[17] While there have been a number of positive nonrandomized studies and a few with wait-list comparison-group studies,[2] there have been no well-designed randomized controlled trials. The potential side effects are the demand of a good deal of time, the expense, and the conflicts between parent and child over compliance.

■ Sensory Integration

Sensory integration was developed by Dr. Jean Ayres[16] and is based on the theory that improvement in the ability to integrate the senses improves the ability to behave and pay attention. It consists of exercises to improve the integration of the senses. While there have been a number of positive nonrandomized or methodologically flawed studies, there are no randomized control trials demonstrating its efficacy.[12] As with biofeedback, the potential side effects are the demand of a good deal of time, the expense, and the conflicts between parent and child over compliance.

■ Auditory Training

Auditory training is based on the theory that improved auditory integration will improve learning and attention.[15] The training consists of auditory desensitization, stimulation, and listening training. There have been no rigorous studies to assess its efficacy and, as with the two previous therapies, the potential side effects are the demand of a good deal of time, the expense, and the conflicts between parent and child over compliance.[11]

The choice of an alternative therapy is usually based upon the belief that a particular therapy is working or will work. While it is always important to be honest and provide accurate information about a particular therapy, it may be counterproductive to try to convince a parent with a strong belief about the lack of scientific evidence for their particular preferred therapy. It is better to maintain a good working relationship since the families frequently require additional interventions. It helps to be a good listener and to assist the parent in assessing whether the intervention is working for their child. Finally, there is no reason that medical treatments cannot be combined with the approaches or supplements mentioned previously. For example, some families may choose to use EEG biofeedback, zinc, and/or omega-3 fatty acids in association with stimulants. A search for drug interactions between the stimulants and the supplements included in this chapter did not identify any significant interactions.

REFERENCES

1. Feingold B. *Why Your Child Is Hyperactive*. New York, NY: Random House; 1975.
2. Rojas NL, Chan E. Old and new controversies in the alternative treatment of attention-deficit hyperactivity disorder. *Ment Retard Dev Disabil Res Rev*. 2005;11:116-130.
3. McCann D, Barrett A, Cooper A, et al. Food additives and hyperactive behaviour in 3-year-old and 8/9-year-old children in the community: a randomised, double-blinded, placebo-controlled trial. *Lancet*. 2007;370:1560-1567.
4. Breakey J. The role of diet and behaviour in childhood. *J Paediatr Child Health*. 1997;33:190-194.
5. Wolraich, ML. Attention Deficit Hyperactivity Disorder: Current Diagnosis and Treatment. Presented at: 55th Annual Meeting of the American Academy of Pediatrics; October 28, 2000; Chicago, IL. Available at: http://medscape.com/viewarticle/420198. Accessed March 30, 2009.
6. Wolraich ML, Wilson DB, White JW. The effect of sugar on behavior or cognition in children. A meta-analysis. *JAMA*. 1995;274:1617-1621.
7. Chan E. Complementary and alternative medicine. In: Wolraich M, Dworkin PH, Drotar DD, Perrin EC, eds. *Developmental-Behavioral Pediatrics: Evidence and Practice*. Philadelphia, PA: Mosby; 2008.
8. Mitchell EA, Aman MG, Turbott SH, Manku M. Clinical characteristics and serum essential fatty acid levels in hyperactive children. *Clin Pediatr (Phila)*. 1987;26:406-411.
9. Stevens LJ, Zentall SS, Deck JL, et al. Essential fatty acid metabolism in boys with attention-deficit hyperactivity disorder. *Am J Clin Nutr*. 1995;62:761-768.
10. Voigt RG, Llorente AM, Jensen CL, Fraley JK, Berretta MC, Heird WC. A randomized, double-blind, placebo-controlled trial of docosahexaenoic acid supplementation in children with attention-deficit/hyperactivity disorder. *J Pediatr*. 2001;139:189-196.
11. Hirayama S, Hamazaki T, Terasawa K. Effect of docosahexaenoic acid-containing food administration on symptoms of attention-deficit/hyperactivity disorder—a placebo-controlled double-blind study. *Eur J Clin Nutr*. 2004;58:467-473.
12. Richardson AJ, Puri BK. A randomized double-blind, placebo-controlled study of the effects of supplementation with highly unsaturated fatty acids on ADHD-related symptoms in children with specific learning difficulties. *Prog Neuropsychopharmacol Biol Psychiatry*. 2002;26:233-239.

13. Arnold LE, Christopher J, Huestis RD, Smeltzer DJ. Megavitamins for minimal brain dysfunction. A placebo-controlled study. *JAMA*. 1978;240:2642-2643.

14. Haslam RH, Dalby JT, Rademaker AW. Effects of megavitamin therapy on children with attention deficit disorders. *Pediatrics*. 1984;74:103-111.

15. Baumgaertel A. Alternative and controversial treatments for attention-deficit/hyperactivity disorder. *Pediatr Clin North Am*. 1999;46:977-992.

16. Goldstein S, Goldstein M. *Managing Attention Deficit Hyperactivity Disorder in Children: A Guide for Practitioners*. 2nd ed. Hoboken, NJ: John Wiley and Sons Inc; 1998.

17. Lubar JO, Lubar JF. Electroencephalographic biofeedback of SMR and beta for treatment of attention deficit disorders in a clinical setting. *Biofeedback Self Regul*. 1984;9:1-23.

8 Substance-Abuse Disorders and Issues Related to ADHD

Substance use and abuse and their relationship to ADHD are important issues for the clinician to understand because many misconceptions are common in the public. Many people have fears about using ADHD medication because of the risk of substance abuse of stimulants or the concern that the use of ADHD medication will increase the risk of developing a substance-abuse problem. This chapter will address these issues, review the data on SUD and ADHD, and offer guidelines for evaluation and treatment of individuals with both disorders.

As described in Chapter 2, *Etiology, Prevalence, and Long-Term Outcomes*, the prevalence rates of ADHD among adolescents is in the range of 2.2% to 9.9%.[1,2] The prevalence of SUD gradually increases from the age of 14 (7%) to the age of 21 (25%).[3] Among the 12- to 17-year-old age group, 9% met criteria for an SUD or dependence diagnosis in the past year; 6% met criteria for an alcohol diagnosis; and 4%, for cannabis abuse or dependence.[3] Approximately 14.4% of children aged 12 to 17 years reported use of a tobacco product in the past month.[3]

Overlap Between ADHD and SUD

Since both ADHD and SUD are common conditions, they would be anticipated to have a fair amount of overlap. However, the actual amount of overlap exceeds what would be expected based upon a random distribution. For example, several epidemiologic studies have found that between one fourth and one third of substance-abusing adolescents meet diagnostic criteria for ADHD.[4-6] In a study of juvenile offenders, 23% of those with SUD were found to have ADHD, while none of those without SUD had ADHD.[7] A retrospective study of adults found that SUD symptoms had an earlier onset among adults with ADHD in comparison to controls. This finding was independent of other psychiatric comorbidity.[8]

Prospective studies have also found this association. Lynskey and Fergusson found a linear relationship between ADHD symptoms in 8 year olds and rates of illicit drug use in 15 year olds.[9] However, this association was explained by the correlation between CD and ADHD.[9] Similar results have been found by Disney and colleagues in a large community study of adolescent twins and by Greenbaum and associates in a clinic population.[10,11] A large longitudinal study has also shown the close association of SUD with ADHD and CD.[12] This study demonstrated that ADHD per se is not a significant independent risk factor for SUD among adolescents, ie, the majority of risk accrues to the comorbid factor of CD.

When reviewing the adult literature, it is clear that adults with ADHD show significant rates of SUD.[13] A comprehensive review by Wilens and coworkers reported rates of alcohol abuse or dependence of 17% to 45% and rates of 9% to 30% for drug abuse or dependence among adults with ADHD.[14] The prevalence of SUD in adults with ADHD is much higher than that seen in populations of adolescents. This may be explained by the fact that the peak age of onset of SUD among those with ADHD is in the early 20s.[15]

Research in adults seeking substance-abuse treatment shows higher than expected rates of ADHD.[16-18] For example, Goodwin and colleagues found much higher rates of childhood ADHD among Danish adoptees with alcoholism than among those without alcoholism.[19] Schubiner and colleagues found a 24% prevalence rate of ADHD (ie, symptoms dating back to childhood and persisting into adulthood) among 201 adults seeking treatment for drug and/or alcohol abuse.[20] The rates of ADHD were higher among men (29%) than among women (19%).[20]

The overall severity of SUD has been found to be increased in those with ADHD. Both Wilens and Carroll reported that ADHD is associated with earlier onset of SUD symptomatology.[8,16] Carroll also reported that those with ADHD had more frequent and more severe cocaine use, while Schubiner and colleagues reported more motor vehicle accidents and prior treatment episodes for SUD in the ADHD subgroup.[18] To date, the literature does not show evidence of preferential abuse of cocaine or stimulants among individuals with ADHD. A study by Biederman and coworkers indicated that marijuana is the most commonly abused drug after alcohol, both in individuals with and in those without ADHD.[20]

Factors Predictive of SUD Among Those With ADHD

In a longitudinal study over 2 decades, Mannuza and colleagues documented the importance of CD as a risk factor for SUD among those with ADHD.[21] Barkley found that adolescents with ADHD without CD did not have higher rates of SUD than did the control group without ADHD.[22] Flory and colleagues found that the combination of ADHD and CD was predictive of higher symptoms of both marijuana and other illicit use than was either ADHD alone or CD alone.[23] Thus the interaction between ADHD and CD appears to be one of the more important variables in evaluating and treating adolescents with SUD. For example, Loeber and associates found that the most adverse outcomes occurred in those with ADHD plus CD as compared with either disorder alone.[24] Conversely, Molina and colleagues found that the severity of adolescent alcohol use disorder was primarily dependent on the presence of CD and the severity of CD, rather than on the combination of ADHD and CD.[25]

In addition to CD, bipolar disorder also confers an increased risk of SUD among those with ADHD as well as among those without ADHD.[26,27] This risk persists even after controlling for comorbid CD. This finding is important, given some evidence that treatment of bipolar disorder may help to improve overall functioning and reduce substance abuse.[28]

While SUD in ADHD adolescents appears to be primarily accounted for by the presence of comorbid CD or bipolar disorder, emerging data suggest that SUD is more prevalent in ADHD adults even if these comorbid features are absent.[20]

The prognosis of those with SUD may be affected by the presence of ADHD. Wilens and colleagues reported that rates of remission and the duration of SUD prior to remission were both significantly more in individuals with ADHD in comparison with controls.[29] Carroll and associates and Whitmore and colleagues documented similar findings in adults and adolescents, respectively.[16,30]

From a developmental and psychological viewpoint, there are several potential reasons for an increased risk of SUD among individuals with ADHD. Neuropsychological dysfunctions are considered to be prevalent to a large degree among both children and adults with ADHD.[31] Executive function deficits go hand in hand with inattention, and deficits such as inability to inhibit responses also impact other executive controls. Therefore, behavioral controls may not be optimal.[31] Impulsive risk-taking behaviors among early adolescents may include drug and alcohol use which puts them at higher risk for long-term use.[32,33] Approximately 30% of individuals with ADHD have comorbid learning disorders, and these deficits make academic failure more likely.[31] There is some evidence to suggest that demoralization due to underachievement and failure can lead to SUD.[34]

Screening and Assessment

It is of critical importance to screen for substance use and SUD in each adolescent who presents for assessment and/or treatment for ADHD. The majority of adolescents have experimented with tobacco, alcohol, marijuana, and other drugs. The clinician should ask each adolescent about the quantity and frequency of use, the presence of adverse consequences of use, and the adolescent's attitude toward use. This evaluation is necessary to determine whether the adolescent is using one or more substances, what effects substance use has on the adolescent's psychosocial functioning, and whether the problem fits diagnostic criteria for substance abuse or dependence. **Figure 8.1** presents an algorithm for the assessment and treatment of substance abuse.

The diagnosis of ADHD in individuals who present with SUD can often be difficult. The current symptoms of SUD may obscure the diagnosis of ADHD, in part because it may be difficult to differentiate drug-induced

FIGURE 8.1 — Algorithm for Assessment and Treatment of Substance Abuse

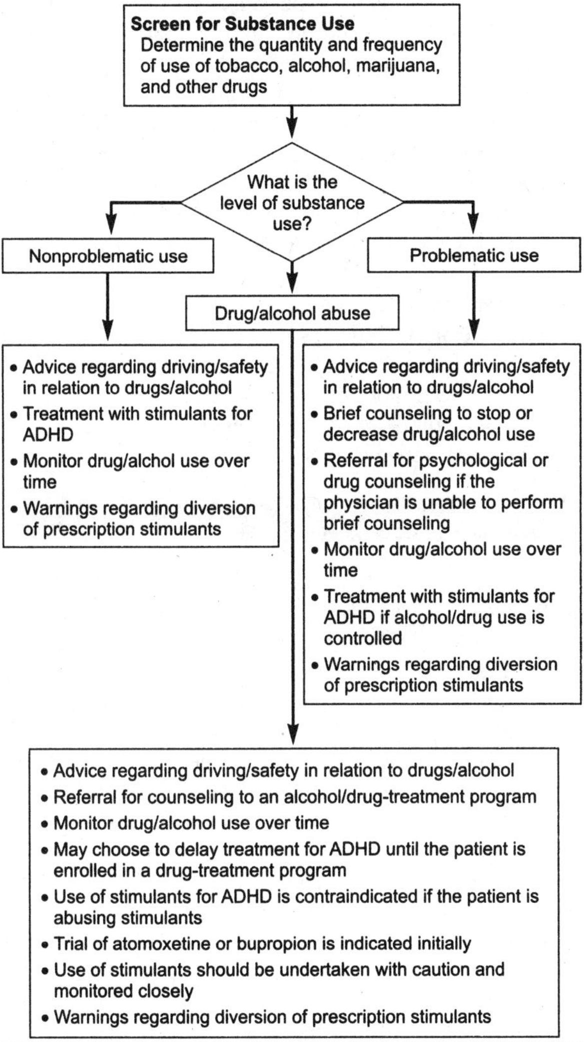

ADHD symptoms from those of their baseline cognitive status. Hyperactivity, agitation, impulsivity, and attentional difficulties may also be caused by withdrawal from various substances. Caution should be taken with drug-seeking individuals with SUD who may feign ADHD symptoms or history and insist on stimulant treatment. A recent set of guidelines for the diagnosis of ADHD in patients with a history of SUD has been published.[35]

It is also important to identify and monitor the level of substance use or abuse that has occurred or is occurring in an adolescent or adult already diagnosed with ADHD. The ADHD treatment can vary significantly, depending on this differentiation. The guidelines for use, abuse, and dependence are included as part of **Table 8.1** and should be used for accurate diagnoses. The type of substances abused is also important, since patients with a history of prescription stimulant abuse or dependence are at higher risk for a recurrence if prescribed stimulant medications.

Treatment

Two well-designed studies have considered the issue of medication treatment for patients with coexisting ADHD and SUD. Schubiner and colleagues performed the first randomized, controlled trial of methylphenidate in patients with ADHD and active cocaine dependence.[36] Levin and colleagues conducted a similar trial, and both studies found that the use of methylphenidate in this high-risk population was quite safe.[37] However, the efficacy of methylphenidate in reducing cocaine use was relatively low. These studies suggest that it is relatively safe to treat patients for ADHD even if they are active users of cocaine and other substances of abuse. However, in order to have a significant impact on their SUD, it is likely that coordinated and intensive efforts will be required.

Despite the fact that there is a paucity of research data, some guidelines have been published for the treatment of co-occurring ADHD and SUD.[38] A set of guidelines developed by Dr. Schubiner is shown in **Table 8.1**. For those adolescents and adults who do not use or abuse alcohol or drugs, treatment with usual medications (typically stimulants as first-line agents) is recommended.

In addition, advice regarding safety and driving, warnings regarding diversion of prescription medications, and monitoring use over time is recommended as described in Chapter 5, *Medication Treatment*. For those with problematic use, but not abuse, similar recommendations usually suffice, but providers should engage in brief counseling to decrease alcohol and/or drug use and minimize harm associated with such use, eg, reduce drinking and driving. Alternatively, a referral to someone who can perform this type of counseling can be done. For those patients with alcohol or drug abuse, a referral to a substance-abuse treatment program is indicated, although the provider may choose to prescribe medications for ADHD as well. In this situation, a trial of atomoxetine or bupropion may be indicated in lieu of stimulant treatment, although some physicians may choose to use stimulant medications under carefully supervised conditions. For patients with alcohol or drug dependence, most providers would require the patient to participate in a substance-abuse treatment program for several weeks prior to the initiation of ADHD medications. Similar guidelines to those for substance abuse would apply regarding which medications to use, although as mentioned, those with a history of stimulant abuse should not be prescribed stimulant medications unless very carefully monitored.

Diversion of Stimulant Medications

Diversion and misuse of prescribed medications is common, particularly in high school and college students. In a 2006 study,[39] almost half of the students had received a prescription for a scheduled medication in their lifetime; and a third had received such a prescription in the past year. Opioid analgesics were the most widely prescribed and the most widely abused. Stimulant and sedative or anxiety medications had lower rates of diversion. In a Canadian survey of 13,549 junior/senior high school students, 15% (of the 5.3% who were prescribed stimulants) reported having given away some of their medication; 7% having sold some of their medication; and 4%, having experienced theft of their medication.[40] In a recent review of stimulant diversion and misuse,[41]

TABLE 8.1 — Levels of Substance Use and Abuse and Suggested Management Approaches

Nonproblematic Drug/Alcohol Use[a]
- Advice regarding driving/safety in relation to drugs/alcohol
- Treatment with stimulants for ADHD
- Monitor drug/alcohol use over time
- Warnings regarding diversion of prescription stimulants

Problematic Drug/Alcohol Use[b]
- Advice regarding driving/safety in relation to drugs/alcohol
- Brief counseling to stop or decrease drug/alcohol use
- Referral for psychological or drug counseling if the physician is unable to perform brief counseling
- Monitor drug/alcohol use over time
- Treatment with stimulants for ADHD if alcohol/drug use is controlled
- Warnings regarding diversion of prescription stimulants

Drug/Alcohol Abuse[c]
- Advice regarding driving/safety in relation to drugs/alcohol
- Referral for counseling to an alcohol/drug-treatment program
- Monitor drug/alcohol use over time
- Treatment with stimulants for ADHD may be undertaken cautiously and monitored closely, but a trial of atomoxetine or bupropion may be indicated
- Warnings regarding diversion of prescription stimulants

Drug/Alcohol Dependence[d]
- Advice regarding driving/safety in relation to drugs/alcohol
- Referral for counseling to an alcohol/drug-treatment program
- Monitor drug/alcohol use over time
- May choose to delay treatment for ADHD until the patient is enrolled in a drug-treatment program
- Use of stimulants for ADHD is contraindicated if the patient is abusing prescription stimulants
- A trial of atomoxetine or bupropion is indicated initially
- Use of stimulants should be undertaken with caution and monitored closely
- Warnings regarding diversion of prescription stimulants

Continued

[a] Defined by any use of alcohol or drugs during the past 12 months with 0-1 alcohol- or drug-related negative consequences (accident, arrest, injury, altercation, interpersonal problem, school problem).

[b] Defined by 2 or more reported alcohol- or drug-related negative consequences within the past 12 months, but no diagnosis of abuse or dependence.

[c] *DSM-IV* criteria include one of the following in the past 12 months: recurrent alcohol or substance use leading to failures at work, at school, or at home, recurrent use leading to legal problems, recurrent use in unsafe situations (eg, driving), and/or continued use despite one of the above problems.

[d] *DSM-IV* criteria include 3 of the following: tolerance, withdrawal symptoms, using more than intended, persistent desire and/or unsuccessful attempts to decrease use, spending a great deal of time using, failure at work, school, or home, and continued use despite being aware of the above problems.

rates of nonprescribed stimulant use were reported to be from 5% to 9% in grade school– and high school–age children and 5% to 35% in college-age individuals. Rates of diversion ranged from 16% to 29% of students with stimulant prescriptions who were asked to give, sell, or trade their medications. However, in a comprehensive, population-based survey of >50,000 individuals, only 2.6% of individuals aged 12 to 17 years of age reported ever having misused an ADHD medication.[42]

Most important, the prevalence of stimulant abuse or dependence among adolescents or young adults with a history of ADHD and therapeutic stimulant use is very low.[43] Overall, diversion is relatively common, but not epidemic among adolescents.

In the absence of clear evidence of ongoing diversion or clear high-risk situations (eg, family member with an active SUD, antisocial personality disorder), the threat of diversion should not be, in and of itself, a reason for withholding or not using stimulant medications. Rather, the clinician should always evaluate the risk factors for diversion and stimulant abuse and set up a clear plan of control and administration of the stimulant (or other) medication. **Table 8.2** offers some guidelines for avoiding and recognizing diversion, misuse, and abuse of stimulant medications. It is generally considered helpful to prescribe longer-acting medications, which appear to have

TABLE 8.2 — Precautions to Avoid Abuse of Stimulants and Red Flags for Misuse or Diversion

Precautions to Avoid Abuse of Stimulants

- Limit and keep track of pills and prescriptions
- Discuss potential cardiac risks for people who have not been cleared to take stimulants
- Frequent patient visits
- Use of long-acting preparations
- Emphasis to patient to take medications regularly, not on an as-needed basis
- Discussion with patient regarding safe storage and avoidance of advertising medications

Red Flags for Misuse or Diversion

- Demands for immediate-release compounds
- Repeated running out of medications in a month
- Frequent lost prescriptions
- Continuously escalating doses
- Symptoms of psychosis, or unpredictable or irrational behavior
- Signs associated with heavier-than-prescribed use (palpitations, tachycardia, hypertension, weight loss)

a lower risk of abuse and misuse in comparison to the shorter-acting preparations. For example, OROS–methylphenidate is difficult to use via a nasal or intravenous route and lisdexamfetamine has very slow conversion to an active agent via these routes.

REFERENCES

1. Skounti M, Philalithis A, Galanakis E. Variations in prevalence of attention deficit hyperactivity disorder worldwide. *Eur J Pediatr.* 2007;166:117-123.
2. Smalley S, McGough JJ, Moilanen IK, et al. Prevalence and psychiatric comorbidity of attention-deficit/hyperactivity disorder in an adolescent Finnish population. *J Am Acad Child Adolesc Psychiatry.* 2007;46:1575-1583.
3. Substance Abuse and Mental Health Services Administration (SAMHSA). Results from the 2005 National Household Survey on Drug Use and Health: National Findings (NSDUH). http://www.oas.samhsa.gov/nsduh/2k5nsduh/2k5Results.htm#TOC. Accessed March 30, 2009.
4. Thompson LL, Riggs PD, Mikulich SK, Crowley TJ. Contribution of ADHD symptoms to substance problems and delinquency in conduct-disordered adolescents. *J Abnorm Child Psychol.* 1996;24:325-347.
5. Winters K. Clinical considerations in the assessment of adolescent chemical dependency. *J Adolesc Chem Depend.* 1990:21-49.
6. DeMilio L. Psychiatric syndromes in adolescent substance abusers. *Am J Psychiatry.* 1989;146:1212-1214.
7. Milin R, Halikas JA, Meller JE, Morse C. Psychopathology among substance abusing juvenile offenders. *J Am Acad Child Adolesc Psychiatry*. 1991;30:569-574.
8. Wilens TE, Biederman J, Mick E, Faraone SV, Spencer T. Attention deficit hyperactivity disorder (ADHD) is associated with early onset substance use disorders. *J Nerv Ment Dis*. 1997;185:475-482.
9. Lynskey MT, Fergusson DM. Childhood conduct problems, attention deficit behaviors, and adolescent alcohol, tobacco, and illicit drug use. *J Abnorm Child Psychol*. 1995;23:281-302.
10. Disney ER, Elkins IJ, McGue M, Iacono WG. Effects of ADHD, conduct disorder, and gender on substance use and abuse in adolescence. *Am J Psychiatry*. 1999;156:1515-1521.
11. Greenbaum PE, Prange ME, Friedman RM, Silver SE. Substance abuse prevalence and comorbidity with other psychiatric disorders among adolescents with severe emotional disturbances. *J Am Acad Child Adolesc Psychiatry*. 1991;30:575-583.
12. Milberger S, Biederman J, Faraone SV, Wilens T, Chu MP. Associations between ADHD and psychoactive substance use disorders. Findings from a longitudinal study of high-risk siblings of ADHD children. *Am J Addict.* 1997;6:318-329.

13. Shekim WO, Asarnow RF, Hess E, Zaucha K, Wheeler N. A clinical and demographic profile of a sample of adults with attention deficit hyperactivity disorder, residual state. *Compr Psychiatry.* 1990;31:416-425.

14. Wilens TE, Spencer TJ, Biederman J. Are attention-deficit hyperactivity disorder and the psychoactive substance use disorders really related? *Harv Rev Psychiatry.* 1995;3:160-162.

15. Biederman J, Wilens TE, Mick E, Faraone SV, Spencer T. Does attention-deficit hyperactivity disorder impact the developmental course of drug and alcohol abuse and dependence? *Biol Psychiatry.* 1998;44:269-273.

16. Carroll KM, Rounsaville BJ. History and significance of childhood attention deficit disorder in treatment-seeking cocaine abusers. *Compr Psychiatry.* 1993;34:75-82.

17. Levin FR, Evans SM, Kleber HD. Prevalence of adult attention-deficit hyperactivity disorder among cocaine abusers seeking treatment. *Drug Alcohol Depend.* 1998;52:15-25.

18. Schubiner H, Tzelepis A, Milberger S, et al. Prevalence of attention-deficit/hyperactivity disorder and conduct disorder among substance abusers. *J Clin Psychiatry.* 2000;61:244-251.

19. Goodwin DW, Schulsinger F, Hermansen L, Guze SB, Winokur G. Alcoholism and the hyperactive child syndrome. *J Nerv Ment Dis.* 1975;160:349-353.

20. Biederman J, Wilens T, Mick E, Milberger S, Spencer TJ, Faraone SV. Psychoactive substance use disorders in adults with attention deficit hyperactivity disorder (ADHD): effects of ADHD and psychiatric comorbidity. *Am J Psychiatry.* 1995;152:1652-1658.

21. Mannuzza S, Klein RG, Bonagura N, Malloy P, Giampino TL, Addalli KA. Hyperactive boys almost grown up. V. Replication of psychiatric status. *Arch Gen Psychiatry.* 1991;48:77-83.

22. Barkley R. *Attention Deficit Hyperactivity Disorder: A Handbook for Diagnosis and Treatment.* 2nd ed. New York, NY: The Guilford Press; 1998.

23. Flory K, Milich R, Lynam DR, Leukefeld C, Clayton R. Relation between childhood disruptive behavior disorders and substance use and dependence symptoms in young adulthood: individuals with symptoms of attention-deficit/hyperactivity disorder and conduct disorder are uniquely at risk. *Psychol Addict Behav.* 2003;17:151-158.

24. Loeber R, Brinthaupt VP, Green SM. Attention deficits, impulsivity, and hyperactivity with or without conduct problems: relationships to delinquency and unique contextual factors. In: McMahon RJ, Peters RD, eds. *Behavior Disorders of Adolescence: Research, Intervention, and Policy in Clinical and School Settings.* New York, NY: Plenum Press; 1990:39-61.

25. Molina BS, Bukstein OG, Lynch KG. Attention-deficit/hyperactivity disorder and conduct disorder symptomatology in adolescents with alcohol use disorder. *Psychol Addict Behav*. 2002;16:161-164.

26. Biederman J, Wilens T, Mick E, et al. Is ADHD a risk factor for psychoactive substance use disorders? Findings from a four-year prospective follow-up study. *J Am Acad Child Adolesc Psychiatry*. 1997;36:21-29.

27. Wilens TE, Biederman J, Millstein RB, Wozniak J, Hahesy AL, Spencer TJ. Risk for substance use disorders in youths with child- and adolescent-onset bipolar disorder. *J Am Acad Child Adolesc Psychiatry*. 1999;38:680-685.

28. Geller B, Cooper TB, Sun K, et al. Double-blind and placebo-controlled study of lithium for adolescent bipolar disorders with secondary substance dependency. *J Am Acad Child Adolesc Psychiatry*. 1998;37:171-178.

29. Wilens TE, Biederman J, Mick E. Does ADHD affect the course of substance abuse? Findings from a sample of adults with and without ADHD. *Am J Addict*. 1998;7:156-163.

30. Whitmore EA, Mikulich SK, Thompson LL, Riggs PD, Aarons GA, Crowley TJ. Influences on adolescent substance dependence: conduct disorder, depression, attention deficit hyperactivity disorder, and gender. *Drug Alcohol Depend*. 1997;47:87-97.

31. Seidman LJ, Doyle A, Fried R, Valera E, Crum K, Matthews L. Neuropsychological function in adults with attention-deficit/hyperactivity disorder. *Psychiatr Clin North Am*. 2004;27:261-282.

32. Kandel DB, Logan JA. Patterns of drug use from adolescence to young adulthood: I. Periods of risk for initiation, continued use, and discontinuation. *Am J Public Health*. 1984;74:660-666.

33. Yamaguchi K, Kandel DB. Patterns of drug use from adolescence to young adulthood: III. Predictors of progression. *Am J Public Health*. 1984;74:673-681.

34. Mannuzza S, Klein RG, Konig PH, Giampino TL. Hyperactive boys almost grown up. IV. Criminality and its relationship to psychiatric status. *Arch Gen Psychiatry*. 1989;46:1073-1079.

35. Levin FR. Diagnosing attention-deficit/hyperactivity disorder in patients with substance use disorders. *J Clin Psychiatry*. 2007;68(suppl 11):9-14.

36. Schubiner H, Saules KK, Arfken CL, et al. Double-blind placebo-controlled trial of methylphenidate in the treatment of adult ADHD patients with comorbid cocaine dependence. *Exp Clin Psychopharmacol*. 2002;10:286-294.

37. Levin FR, Evans SM, Brooks DJ, Garawi F. Treatment of cocaine dependent treatment seekers with adult ADHD: double-blind comparison of methylphenidate and placebo. *Drug Alcohol Depend*. 2007;87:20-29.

38. Mariani JJ, Levin FR. Treatment strategies for co-occurring ADHD and substance use disorders. *Am J Addict.* 2007;16(suppl 1):45-54.

39. Boyd CJ, Esteban McCabe S, Teter CJ. Medical and nonmedical use of prescription pain medication by youth in a Detroit-area public school district. *Drug Alcohol Depend.* 2006;81:37-45.

40. Poulin C. Medical and nonmedical stimulant use among adolescents: from sanctioned to unsanctioned use. *CMAJ.* 2001;165:1039-1044.

41. Wilens TE, Adler LA, Adams J, et al. Misuse and diversion of stimulants prescribed for ADHD: a systematic review of the literature. *J Am Acad Child Adolesc Psychiatry.* 2008;47:21-31.

42. Kroutil LA, Van Brunt DL, Herman-Stahl MA, Heller DC, Bray RM, Penne MA. Nonmedical use of prescription stimulants in the United States. *Drug Alcohol Depend.* 2006;84:135-143.

43. Kollins SH. Abuse liability of medications used to treat attention-deficit/hyperactivity disorder (ADHD). *Am J Addict.* 2007;16(suppl 1):35-42.

9 Appendices

The following rating scale and assessments are contained in this chapter:

- Appendix 1—Vanderbilt Parent-Assessment Scale
- Appendix 2—Vanderbilt Parent-Assessment Follow-Up
- Apppendix 3—Vanderbilt Teacher-Assessment Scale
- Appendix 4—Vanderbilt Teacher-Assessment Follow-Up
- Appendix 5—Pittsburgh Side Effects–Rating Scale.

APPENDIX 1 — Vanderbilt Parent-Assessment Scale

Date ______________ Child's Name ________________________________ Date of Birth ______________

Parent's Name ________________________________

Each rating should be considered in the context of what is appropriate for the age of your child.

This evaluation is based on a time when the child… ☐ was on medication. ☐ was not on medication.

Symptoms	Never	Occasionally	Often	Very Often
1. Does not pay attention to detail or makes careless mistakes with, for example, homework	0	1	2	3
2. Has difficulty keeping attention on what needs to be done	0	1	2	3
3. Does not seem to listen when spoken to directly	0	1	2	3
4. Does not follow through when given directions and fails to finish activities (not due to refusal or misunderstanding)	0	1	2	3
5. Has difficulty organizing tasks and activities	0	1	2	3
6. Avoids, dislikes, or does not want to start tasks that require ongoing mental effort	0	1	2	3
7. Loses things necessary for tasks or activities (toys, assignments, pencils, or books)	0	1	2	3
8. Is easily distracted by noises or other stimuli	0	1	2	3
9. Is forgetful in daily activities	0	1	2	3

10. Fidgets with hands or feet or squirms in seat	0	1	2	3
11. Leaves seat when remaining seated is expected	0	1	2	3
12. Runs about or climbs too much when remaining seated is expected	0	1	2	3
13. Has difficulty playing or beginning quiet play activities	0	1	2	3
14. Is “on the go” or often acts as if “driven by a motor”	0	1	2	3
15. Talks too much	0	1	2	3
16. Blurts out answers before questions have been completed	0	1	2	3
17. Has difficulty waiting his or her turn	0	1	2	3
18. Interrupts or intrudes in others’ conversations and/or activities	0	1	2	3
19. Argues with adults	0	1	2	3
20. Loses temper	0	1	2	3
21. Actively defies or refuses to go along with adults’ requests or rules	0	1	2	3
22. Deliberately annoys people	0	1	2	3
23. Blames others for his or her mistakes or misbehaviors	0	1	2	3
24. Is touchy or easily annoyed by others	0	1	2	3
25. Is angry or resentful	0	1	2	3
26. Is spiteful and wants to get even	0	1	2	3
27. Bullies, threatens, or intimidates others	0	1	2	3
28. Starts physical fights	0	1	2	3
29. Lies to get out of trouble or to avoid obligations (ie, “cons” others)	0	1	2	3

Continued

APPENDIX 1 — *Continued*

Symptoms	Never	Occasionally	Often	Very Often
30. Is truant from school (skips school) without permission	0	1	2	3
31. Is physically cruel to people	0	1	2	3
32. Has stolen things that have value	0	1	2	3
33. Deliberately destroys others' property	0	1	2	3
34. Has used a weapon that can cause serious harm (bat, knife, brick, gun)	0	1	2	3
35. Is physically cruel to animals	0	1	2	3
36. Has deliberately set fires to cause damage	0	1	2	3
37. Has broken into someone else's home, business, or car	0	1	2	3
38. Has stayed out at night without permission	0	1	2	3
39. Has run away from home overnight	0	1	2	3
40. Has forced someone into sexual activity	0	1	2	3
41. Is fearful, anxious, or worried	0	1	2	3
42. Is afraid to try new things for fear of making mistakes	0	1	2	3
43. Feels worthless or inferior	0	1	2	3
44. Blames self for problems, feels guilty	0	1	2	3
45. Feels lonely, unwanted, or unloved; complains "no one loves him/her"	0	1	2	3
46. Is sad, unhappy, or depressed	0	1	2	3
47. Is self-conscious or easily embarrassed	0	1	2	3

Performance	Excellent	Above Average	Average	Somewhat of a Problem	Problematic
48. Overall school performance	1	2	3	4	5
49. Reading	1	2	3	4	5
50. Writing	1	2	3	4	5
51. Mathematics	1	2	3	4	5
52. Relationship with parents	1	2	3	4	5
53. Relationship with siblings	1	2	3	4	5
54. Relationship with peers	1	2	3	4	5
55. Participation in organized activities (eg, teams)	1	2	3	4	5

Scoring Instructions: These are the scoring instructions for the Vanderbilt Evaluation Parent-Rating Scale. These scales should NOT be used alone to make any diagnosis. You must take into consideration information from multiple sources and questionnaires. Scores of 2 or 3 on a single item reflect *often occurring* behaviors.

Inattention (Inattentive Subtype; items 1-9): Must score a 2 or 3 on 6 out of 9 of items 1-9 AND score a 1 or 2 on any 4 of the performance section items.

Hyperactivity/Impulsivity (Hyperactive/Impulsive Subtype; items 10-18): Must score a 2 or 3 on 6 out of 9 of items 10-18 AND score a 1 or 2 on any 8 of the performance section items.

Inattention and Hyperactivity/Impulsivity (Combined Subtype; items 1-9 and 10-18): Must score a 2 or 3 on 6 out of 9 of items 1-9 AND must score a 2 or 3 on 6 out of 9 of items 10-18 AND score a 1 or 2 on any 8 of the performance section items.

Oppositional-Defiant/Conduct Disorder (items 19-28): Must score a 2 or 3 on 3 out of 10 of items 19-28.

Anxiety/Depression (items 29-35): Must score a 2 or 3 on 3 out of 7 of items 29-35.

APPENDIX 2 — Vanderbilt Parent-Assessment Follow-Up

Date ______________ Child's Name ________________________________ Date of Birth ______________

Parent's Name ________________________________

Each rating should be considered in the context of what is appropriate for the age of your child.

This evaluation is based on a time when the child… ☐ was on medication. ☐ was not on medication.

Symptoms	Never	Occasionally	Often	Very Often
1. Does not pay attention to detail or makes careless mistakes with, for example, homework	0	1	2	3
2. Has difficulty keeping attention on what needs to be done	0	1	2	3
3. Does not seem to listen when spoken to directly	0	1	2	3
4. Does not follow through when given directions and fails to finish activities (not due to refusal or misunderstanding)	0	1	2	3
5. Has difficulty organizing tasks and activities	0	1	2	3
6. Avoids, dislikes, or does not want to start tasks that require ongoing mental effort	0	1	2	3
7. Loses things necessary for tasks or activities (toys, assignments, pencils, or books)	0	1	2	3
8. Is easily distracted by noises or other stimuli	0	1	2	3
9. Is forgetful in daily activities	0	1	2	3
10. Fidgets with hands or feet or squirms in seat	0	1	2	3

11. Leaves seat when remaining seated is expected		0	1	2	3
12. Runs about or climbs too much when remaining seated is expected		0	1	2	3
13. Has difficulty playing or beginning quiet play activities		0	1	2	3
14. Is "on the go" or often acts as if "driven by a motor"		0	1	2	3
15. Talks too much		0	1	2	3
16. Blurts out answers before questions have been completed		0	1	2	3
17. Has difficulty waiting his or her turn		0	1	2	3
18. Interrupts or intrudes in others' conversations and/or activities		0	1	2	3

Performance	**Excellent**	**Above Average**	**Average**	**Somewhat of a Problem**	**Problematic**
Academic					
19. Overall school performance	1	2	3	4	5
20. Reading	1	2	3	4	5
21. Writing	1	2	3	4	5
22. Mathematics	1	2	3	4	5
Social					
23. Relationship with parents	1	2	3	4	5
24. Relationship with siblings	1	2	3	4	5
25. Relationship with peers	1	2	3	4	5
26. Participation in organized activities (eg, teams)	1	2	3	4	5

APPENDIX 3 — Vanderbilt Teacher-Assessment Scale

Teacher's Name ______________________ Teacher's Telephone ______________

Child's Name ______________________ Grade ______________

Each rating should be considered in the context of what is appropriate for the age of the child you are rating and should reflect that child's behavior since the beginning of the school year. Please indicate the number of weeks or months you have been able to evaluate the behaviors: ____________

This evaluation is based on a time when the child… ☐ was on medication. ☐ was not on medication.

Symptoms	**Never**	**Occasionally**	**Often**	**Very Often**
1. Fails to give attention to details or makes careless mistakes in schoolwork	0	1	2	3
2. Has difficulty sustaining attention to tasks or activities	0	1	2	3
3. Does not seem to listen when spoken to directly	0	1	2	3
4. Does not follow through on instructions and fails to finish schoolwork (not due to oppositional behavior or failure to understand)	0	1	2	3
5. Has difficulty organizing tasks and activities	0	1	2	3
6. Avoids, dislikes, or does not want to start tasks that require ongoing mental effort	0	1	2	3
7. Loses things necessary for tasks or activities (school assignments, pencils, or books)	0	1	2	3
8. Is easily distracted by extraneous stimuli	0	1	2	3
9. Is forgetful in daily activities	0	1	2	3

10. Fidgets with hands or feet or squirms in seat	0	1	2	3
11. Leaves seat in classroom or in other situations in which remaining seated is expected	0	1	2	3
12. Runs about or climbs excessively in situations in which remaining seated is expected	0	1	2	3
13. Has difficulty playing or engaging in leisure activities quietly	0	1	2	3
14. Is “on the go” or often acts as if “driven by a motor”	0	1	2	3
15. Talks excessively	0	1	2	3
16. Blurts out answers before questions have been completed	0	1	2	3
17. Has difficulty waiting in line	0	1	2	3
18. Interrupts or intrudes in on others (eg, butts into conversations/games)	0	1	2	3
19. Loses temper	0	1	2	3
20. Actively defines or refuses to comply with adults’ requests or rules	0	1	2	3
21. Is angry or resentful	0	1	2	3
22. Is spiteful and vindictive	0	1	2	3
23. Bullies, threatens, or intimidates others	0	1	2	3
24. Initiates physical fights	0	1	2	3
25. Lies to obtain goods for favors or to avoid obligations (eg, “cons” others)	0	1	2	3
26. Is physically cruel to people	0	1	2	3
27. Has stolen items of nontrivial value	0	1	2	3

Continued

APPENDIX 3 — *Continued*

Symptoms	Never	Occasionally	Often	Very Often
28. Deliberately destroys others' property	0	1	2	3
29. Is fearful, anxious, or worried	0	1	2	3
30. Is self-conscious or easily embarrassed	0	1	2	3
31. Is afraid to try new things for fear of making mistakes	0	1	2	3
32. Feels worthless or inferior	0	1	2	3
33. Blames self for problems; feels guilty	0	1	2	3
34. Feels lonely, unwanted, or unloved; complains "no one loves him/her"	0	1	2	3
35. Is sad, unhappy, or depressed	0	1	2	3

Performance	Excellent	Above Average	Average	Somewhat of a Problem	Problematic
36. Reading	1	2	3	4	5
37. Mathematics	1	2	3	4	5
38. Written expression	1	2	3	4	5

Classroom Behavioral Performance

39. Relationship with peers	1	2	3	4	5
40. Following directions	1	2	3	4	5
41. Disrupting class	1	2	3	4	5
42. Assignment completion	1	2	3	4	5
43. Organizational skills	1	2	3	4	5

Scoring Instructions: These are the scoring instructions for the Vanderbilt Evaluation Teacher-Rating Scale. These scales should NOT be used alone to make any diagnosis. You must take into consideration information from multiple sources and questionnaires. Scores of 2 or 3 on a single item reflect often-occurring behaviors.

Inattention (Inattentive Subtype; items 1-9): Must score a 2 or 3 on 6 out of 9 of items 1-9 AND score a 1 or 2 on any 8 of the performance section items.

Hyperactivity/Impulsivity (Hyperactive / Impulsive Subtype; items 10-18): Must score a 2 or 3 on 6 out of 9 of items 10-18 AND score a 1 or 2 on any 8 of the performance section items.

Inattention and Hyperactivity/Impulsivity (Combined Subtype; items 1-9 and 10-18): Must score a 2 or 3 on 6 out of 9 of items 1-9 AND must score a 2 or 3 on 6 out of 9 of items 10-18 AND score a 1 or 2 on any 8 of the performance section items.

Oppositional-Defiant/Conduct Disorder (items 19-28): Must score a 2 or 3 on 3 out of 10 of items 19-28.

Anxiety/Depression (items 29-35): Must score a 2 or 3 on 3 out of 7 of items 29-35.

APPENDIX 4 — Vanderbilt Teacher-Assessment Follow-Up

Teacher's Name__________________ Teacher's Telephone__________ Today's Date_______

Child's Name ________________________________ Grade_______

Each rating should be considered in the context of what is appropriate for the age of the child.

This evaluation is based on a time when the child… ☐ was on medication. ☐ was not on medication.

Symptoms	Never	Occasionally	Often	Very Often
1. Does not pay attention to detail or makes careless mistakes with, for example, homework	0	1	2	3
2. Has difficulty keeping attention on what needs to be done	0	1	2	3
3. Does not seem to listen when spoken to directly	0	1	2	3
4. Does not follow through when given directions and fails to finish activities (not due to refusal or misunderstanding)	0	1	2	3
5. Has difficulty organizing tasks and activities	0	1	2	3
6. Avoids, dislikes, or does not want to start tasks that require ongoing mental effort	0	1	2	3
7. Loses things necessary for tasks or activities (toys, assignments, pencils, or books)	0	1	2	3
8. Is easily distracted by noises or other stimuli	0	1	2	3
9. Is forgetful in daily activities	0	1	2	3
10. Fidgets with hands or feet or squirms in seat	0	1	2	3

11. Leaves seat when remaining seated is expected	0	1	2	3
12. Runs about or climbs too much when remaining seated is expected	0	1	2	3
13. Has difficulty playing or beginning quiet play activities	0	1	2	3
14. Is "on the go" or often acts as if "driven by a motor"	0	1	2	3
15. Talks too much	0	1	2	3
16. Blurts out answers before questions have been completed	0	1	2	3
17. Has difficulty waiting his or her turn	0	1	2	3
18. Interrupts or intrudes in others' conversations and/or activities	0	1	2	3

Performance	**Above Excellent**	**Average**	**Somewhat of a Average**	**Problem**	**Problematic**
19. Reading	1	2	3	4	5
20. Mathematics	1	2	3	4	5
21. Written expression	1	2	3	4	5
22. Relationship with peers	1	2	3	4	5
23. Following direction	1	2	3	4	5
24. Disrupting class	1	2	3	4	5
25. Assignment completion	1	2	3	4	5
26. Organizational skills	1	2	3	4	5

APPENDIX 5 — Pittsburgh Side-Effects–Rating Scale

Instructions: Listed below are several possible negative effects (side effects) that medication may have on an ADHD child. Please read each item carefully and use the boxes to rate the severity of the child's side effects he/she has been on his/her current dose of medication. When requested, or wherever you feel it would be useful for us to know, please describe the side effects that you observed or any other unusual behaviors in the "Comments" section below.

Use the following to assess severity:

None The symptom is not present.

Mild The symptom is present but is not sufficient enough to cause concern to your child, to you, or to his/her friends. Presence of the symptom at this level would NOT be a reason to stop taking the medicine.

Moderate The symptom causes impairment of functioning or social embarrassment to such a degree that the negative impact on social and school performance should be weighed carefully to justify benefit of continuing medication must be considered.

Severe The symptom causes impairment of functioning or social embarrassment to such a degree that the child should not continue to receive this medication or dose of medication as part of current treatment.

	None	Mild	Moderate	Severe
Motor tics—repetitive movements: jerking or twitching (eg, eye blinking-eye opening, facial or mouth twitching, shoulder or arm movements). Please describe: ______________________ ______________________	☐	☐	☐	☐

Buccal-lingual movements: tongue thrusts, jaw clenching, chewing movement besides lip/cheek biting. Please describe: ____________	☐	☐	☐	☐
Picking at skin or fingers, nail biting, lip or cheek chewing. Please describe: ____________	☐	☐	☐	☐
Worried/anxious	☐	☐	☐	☐
Dull, tired, listless	☐	☐	☐	☐
Headaches	☐	☐	☐	☐
Stomach ache	☐	☐	☐	☐
Crabby, irritable	☐	☐	☐	☐
Tearful, sad, depressed	☐	☐	☐	☐
Socially withdrawn (decreased interaction with others)	☐	☐	☐	☐
Hallucinations (sees or hears things that are not there)	☐	☐	☐	☐
Loss of appetite	☐	☐	☐	☐
Trouble sleeping (time went to sleep)	☐	☐	☐	☐

Comments: ____________

9

10 Abbreviations/Acronyms

AACAP	American Academy of Child and Adolescent Psychiatry
AAP	American Academy of Pediatrics
ADD	attention deficit disorder
ADDA	Attention Deficit Disorder Association
ADHA-HI	*DSM-IV* hyperactivity/impulsive symptom cluster
ADHD	attention-deficit/hyperactivity disorder
ADHD-IA	*DSM-IV* inattention symptom cluster
ADHD-RS-IV	Attention-Deficit/Hyperactivity Disorder Rating Scale IV, rated and scored by investigators based on parent reports
AHA	American Heart Association
ANOVA	analysis of variance
ASRS	Adult Self-Rating Scale
BAADS	Brown Adults Attention Disorder Scale
BASC-2	Behavioral Assessment System for Children, 2nd edition
bid	twice daily
CAARS	Conners Adult ADHD Rating Scale
CADS-P	Conner's ADHD/*DSM-IV* rating scale for Parents
CBCL	Child behavior checklist
CD	conduct disorder
CDC	Centers for Disease Control
CGI-I	Dichotomized Clinical Global Impressions–Improvement
CHADD	Children and Adults With Attention-Deficit/Hyperactivity Disorder
CLAM	Conners, Loney, and Milich rating scale
CNS	central nervous system
CPRS-R	Conner's Parent Rating Scale–Revised (hyperactivity subscale)
CTGI	Conner's Teacher Global Index
CTRS-R	Conner's Teacher Rating Scale–Revised (hyperactivity subscale)
DCD	development coordination disorder

DEX	dexamphetamine
DSM	Diagnostic and Statistical Manual of Mental Disorders
ECG	electrocardiogram
EEG	electroencephalogram
EFA	essential fatty acids
FDA	Food and Drug Administration
fMRI	functional magnetic resonance imaging
GAD	generalized anxiety disorder
GI	gastrointestinal
h	hour(s)
HC	hypertrophic cardiomyopathy
HI	hyperactive/impulsive
IA	inattentive
IDEA	Individuals with Disability Education Act
I/O	inattention/overactivity
IEP	individual education plan
IR	immediate-release [formulation]
IY	Incredible Years
LA	long-acting [formulation]
LDX	lisdexamfetamine
LS	least squares [mean score]
MAS XR	mixed amphetamine salts extended-release
MBD	minimal cerebral/brain dysfunction/damage
MPH	methylphenidate
MRI	magnetic resonance imaging
MTA	Multi-Modal Therapy of ADHD
NIMH	National Institute for Mental Health
OCD	obsessive-compulsive disorder
ODD	oppositional defiant disorder
OROS	osmotic-release oral system
OROS MPH	osmotic-release methylphenidate
OT	occupational therapist
PANDAS	pediatric autoimmune neuropsychiatric disorders associated with streptococcal infection
PCIT	parent-child interaction therapy
PERMP	Permanent Product Measure of Performance

PTSD	posttraumatic stress disorder
qd	every day
SAD	separation anxiety disorder
SCD	sudden cardiac death
SKAMP	Swanson, Kotkin, Atkins, M-Flynn, and Pelham rating scale
SKAMP-D	Swanson, Kotkin, Agler, M-Flynn, and Pelham Deportment subscale score
SPECT	single-photon emission computed tomography
SUD	substance use disorder
tid	three times a day
WAIS	Wechsler Adult Intelligence Scale
WISC-IV	Wechsler Intelligence Scale for Children, 4th edition

Note: Page numbers in *italics* indicate figures.
Page numbers followed by a "t" indicate tables.

1-2-3 Magic: Effective Discipline for Children (Phelan), 100t
Academic performance, 20, 33-35
Accommodations, academic or employment, 54-55, 105-106, 109
ADD (attention-deficit disorder), 12
 with or without hyperactivity (*DSM-III*), *11*, 12
 organizations and web sites, 56
ADD Warehouse, 56
ADDA (web site), 56
Adderall, Adderall XR, 66t, 81. See also *Amphetamines.*
 cardiac side effects and, 78-79
 duration of action, *80*, 81
 efficacy and safety, 81, *82*
Additives, food, 111-112
ADHD (attention-deficit/hyperactivity disorder)
 controversy about, 13
 core symptoms, 24t
 destigmatizing, 49, 55-56
 etiology of, 15-16
 history of, 9-12, *11*
 impact of, 9, 20-21
 introduction to, 9-14
 long-term outcomes, 20-21
 myths about (and corrections), 9-12
 prevalence of, 12, 16-20, *18*, 119
 school services for, 105-107
 "subsyndromal," 29-30
 subtypes, *11*, 12, 23, 24t, 27-28
 support/advocacy groups, 56
 timeline, *11*
Adolescents
 behavioral interventions for, 107-109
 brain development in, 50, 62
 communication with, 107
 comorbid conditions in, 62
 conduct disorder and, 121
 diagnosis in, 24-25, 28-29
  algorithm for, *25*
  difficulties of, 62
 driving (motor vehicle), 52, 94, 125, 126t
 feedback for, 47-49, 107
 medications, 124-125. See also *Medications for ADHD.*
  algorithm for, *93*
  coverage needs, 94
  diversion of, 94, 125-128, 128t

Adolescents, medications *(continued)*
duration of action, 77
efficacy, 62, 81, *82*
response rate, 60
positive reinforcement for, 107
prevalence of ADHD in, 119
rating scales for, 30-31, 30t, 32t
risk-taking behaviors, 52, 122
substance-use/abuse disorders and, 119-122, 125-127
screening for, 122-124, *123*
symptoms in
change with age, 30
continuing into adulthood, 9, 12, 30
core, 24t
transition to adulthood, 50-55
driving, 52
planning for independence, 52-55, 53t
post-high school years, 53-55, 53t
risk-taking behaviors, 52, 122
treatment/management plan for, 50-55, 53t
participation in, 50-51, 62
Adults
behavioral interventions for, 107-109
comorbidities in, 56, 62
diagnosis in, 16, 24-26, *26*, 28-29
management plan for, 55-57
medications. See also *Medications for ADHD.*
algorithm for, *93*
benefit of, 12, 13
duration of action, 77
lisdexamfetamine approval/efficacy for, 83-86, *84-85*, *87*
nonstimulant, 86-88
OROS-MPH approval/efficacy for, 72, *73*
response rate, 60
prevalence rate in, 19
rating scales for, 31-32, 32t
substance-use disorders in, 120-122
symptoms in, 9, 12, 20, 30
Wechsler Adult Intelligence Scale (WAIS), 34
Advocacy groups, 56
Affective disorder, 56
African Americans
ADHD diagnosis in, 20
ADHD prevalence in, 19
ADHD treatment efficacy in, 20
Age
ADHD symptoms and, 9, 12
stimulant medications and, 60-61, 91

Agitation
bupropion and, 90
manic/depressive episodes and, 38t
withdrawal from substance use and, 124
Alcohol
abuse/dependence, 119, 120, 121
fetal exposure to, 15, 41
Algorithms for diagnosis
of ADHD in adults, *26*
of ADHD in children/adolescents, *27*
of substance abuse, *123*
α-Adrenergic medications, 89-90
Alternative treatments for ADHD
alternative medications, 114-115
communicating with patient about, 116
dietary supplements, 113-114
diets, 111-113
exercises and training, 115-116
American Academy of Child and Adolescent Psychiatry (AACAP), 79
American Academy of Pediatrics (AAP)
guidelines for diagnosis, 23-24
recommendation on ECGs, 79
American Heart Association (AHA) recommendations, 78-79
Americans With Disabilities Act, 54, 109
Amphetamine salts, mixed, 66t, 81
efficacy, 81, *82*
vs lisdexamfetamine, 83, *84-85*
Amphetamines, 66t, 79-86. See also *specific amphetamines.*
dextroamphetamine, 66t, 79-80
dosing, 66t, 91
duration of action, 79, 80, *80*
lisdexamfetamine, 66t, 81-86
in medication algorithm, *93*
mixed amphetamine salts, 66t, 81
prodrug (lisdexamfetamine), 81-83
selection of, 91
side effects, 79-80, 81
Anorexia. See also *Appetite suppression.*
α-adrenergic medications and, 90
bupropion and, 90
mixed amphetamine salts and, 81
tricyclic antidepressants and, 89
Antibiotics, 114
Anticholinergic effects, tricyclic antidepressants and, 89
Antidepressants, tricyclic, 59, 89
Antifungal agents, 114-115
Antioxidants, 114
Antisocial personality disorder, 36, 127
Anxiety disorders, 28, 32-33, 39, 56, 62
Apnea, sleep, 32

Appetite suppression. See also *Anorexia.*
amphetamines and, 80, 81
atomoxetine and, 86
lisdexamfetamine and, 86
methylphenidate and, 75
modafinil and, 91
Armed services, career in, 55
Arrhythmias, cardiac, 56, 78
tricyclic antidepressants and, 89
Assessment. See *Diagnosis; Rating scales.*
Atomoxetine (Strattera), 86-88, 94
efficacy, 86, *88*
as first drug of choice, 94
half-life, 86
in medication algorithm, *93*
in substance-use disorders, 126t
Attention-deficit disorder (ADD), *11*, 12, 56
Attention-deficit/hyperactivity disorder. See *ADHD.*
Auditory training, 116
Autism, 28, 32
Ayres, Jean, 115

Barkley rating scale, 31
Behavior-modification training, 99-105
books and web resources, 100t
principle elements of, 104t
programs in, 101t-103t
Behavioral Assessment System for Children, 2nd Edition (BASC-2), 35
Behavioral disorders, other than ADHD, 35-40
Behavioral interventions, 89, 99-105
for adolescents and adults, 107-109
for pre-school children, 62, *92*, 99
Benzedrine, *11*, 59
Biofeedback, 115
Bipolar disorder, 32-33, 36-38, 38t, 62
substance-use disorders and, 121
Birth, premature, 15
Birth trauma, 15
Blood pressure, monitoring, 79, 92
Bradley, C., *11*, 59
Brain
anatomy, 15-16
development, 50, 61, 62
imaging, 16
Brain damage
ADHD and, 10-12, 15-16
minimal cerebral (MBD), 10-12, *11*, 13
Brown, Tom, 32
Brown Adult ADD Scale, 32t

11

Brown Adults Attention Disorder Scale (BAADS), 32
Bupropion (Wellbutrin), 90, 126t

CAARS (Conners Adult ADHD Rating Scale), 31
Candida, 114
Cannabis use/abuse, 119, 121
Cardiac arrhythmias, 56, 78, 89
Cardiac history and evaluation, 78-79
Cardiac side effects, 78-79, 128t
Cars/driving. See *Driving.*
Catapres (clonidine), 89-90
CD. See *Conduct disorder.*
Center for Effective Parenting, 100t
Centers for Disease Control (CDC) study, 19
Central nervous system (CNS). See also *Brain.*
  disorders, ruling out in diagnosis, 32
  mechanisms in ADHD, 15-16
Cerebral metabolic enhancing agents, 115
Cerebral palsy, 32
CHADD (Children and Adults with ADHD), 56, 100, 100t
  parenting program, 101t-103t
Chamomile, 114
Child and Family WebGuide, 100t
Child Behavior Checklist (CBCL), 35
Childhood schizophrenia, 28
Children
  behavioral interventions for, 62, *92*, 99-105
  bipolar disorder symptoms in, 37-38
  brain development in, 61
  core symptoms, 24t
    continuing into adulthood, 9, 12, 30
    monitoring, 91-94
  daily report card (DRC), 107, 108t
  diagnosis in, 16, 23-25, *25*
  diets for ADHD, 111-112
  feedback for, 47-49, 107, 108t
  growth potential/height, 61, 76
  Incredible Years (*IY*) training, 101t
  management plan for, 45-49, 46t, *48*
  medications for. See also *Medications for ADHD.*
    age and, 60-61, 91
    algorithms for, *92*, *93*
    dosing, 91
    nonstimulant medications, 86
    response rates, 60-61, *61*
    safety concerns and recommendations, 61-62, 78-79
    stimulant medications, 35, 60-61, 83
  other behavioral disorders, 35-40
  parent-training programs and, 99-105, 100t, 101t-103t
  positive attention and reinforcement for, 103-105, 104t

Children *(continued)*
  prevalence of substance use disorders, 119
  rating scales for, 30-31, 30t
  sudden cardiac death in, 78, 79
  Wechsler Intelligence Scale for (WISC-IV), 34
Children and Adults with ADHD (CHADD), 56, 100, 100t
  parenting program, 101t-103t
Children's Depression Inventory, 35
Chronic-illness model for ADHD, 45-57, 46t
Cigarettes. See *Nicotine exposure.*
Clinical information systems, 46, 46t
Clinical interview, *25, 26*
Clonidine (Catapres), 89-90
Closed head injuries, 32, 41
CNS. See *Central nervous system.*
Coaching, 99, 107-109
Cocaine use, 120, 121
Cognitive impairments, 32, 33-35
Cognitive therapies, 99
College
  medication coverage needs during, 94
  medication diversion and, 94, 125-127, 128t
  planning for students with ADHD, 53-55, 53t
Communication, 47-49, 57, 107
  about alternative therapies, 116
  about confidentiality, 51
  daily report card, 107, 108t
  destigmatizing ADHD, 49, 55-56
Community resources, 45-46, 46t, 57
Comorbid conditions, 32, 33-41, 56, 62. See also *Substance-use disorders.*
  externalizing conditions, 35-36, 36t
  internalizing conditions, 36-40, 38t
  learning and language disorders, 33-35
  motor disorders/physical conditions, 40-41
  other behavioral disorders, 35-40
  prevalence in ADHD, 33
Concerta. See *OROS-methylphenidate.*
Conduct disorder (CD), 35-36, 37t
  substance-use disorders and, 36, 120, 121
Confidentiality, provider communication about, 51
Conners Rating Scales, 30, 30t, 31
  Adolescent ADD Scale, 32t
  Adolescent ADHD scale, 31
  Adult ADD Scale, 32t
  Adult ADHD Rating Scale (CAARS), 31
  specific medication assessments with
    methylphenidate CD, 69-70, *70*
    mixed amphetamine salts, 81, *82*
    Ritalin LA, 70-71, *71*

11

Conners Rating Scales *(continued)*
  Teacher and Parent Rating Scales, Revised, 30, 30t, 35
Consultants, 46, 47
Controversies about ADHD, 13
Coordination deficits, 31
Coronary heart disease, 56
Counseling, 107-109
  for substance abuse, 125, 126t
Criminal justice department, career in, 55
Cultural differences, 27t
Cytochrome P-450 2D6 pathway, 86

D4 receptor gene (DRD4), 15
Daily report card (DRC), 107, 108t
Daytrana (methylphenidate transdermal patch), 66t
  abuse potential, reduced, 64
  dosing, 66t, 91
  duration of action, *77*
Death, thoughts of
  atomoxetine and, 86
  major depression and, 38t
Decision support, 46, 46t
Depression, 32-33, 36-39, 38t, 62
  bipolar disorder and, 36-38, 38t
  major depressive episode, 36-37, 38t
Desipramine (Norpramin), 89
Destigmatizing ADHD, 49, 55-56
Developmental coordination disorder (DCD), 31, 40-41
Developmental disorders, pervasive, 28, 32
Developmental level, diagnosis and, 23, 28
Dexamphetamine. See *Dextroamphetamine.*
Dexedrine, Dexedrine Spansule, 66t. See also *Dextroamphetamine.*
Dexmethylphenidate (Focalin, Focalin XR), 66t, 73-74
  dosing and pharmacokinetics, 66t, 77
  duration of action, *77*
  efficacy, 73-74, *74*
Dextroamphetamine (Dexedrine, Dexedrine Spansule, Dextrostat), 59, 66t
  dosing and pharmacokinetics, 66t, 80
  duration of action, 79, 80, *80*
  efficacy, 60
  half-life, 79
  safety, 63, 80
  side effects, 79-80
  vs methylphenidate, 65, 67t, 68t
Dextrostat, 66t. See also *Dextroamphetamine.*
Diagnosis of ADHD, 13, 23-43
  AAP guidelines, 23-24
  in adults, 16, 24-27, *26*, 28-29
    algorithm for, *26*

Diagnosis of ADHD *(continued)*
challenges/difficulties in, 16, 17-18, 28-33, 122-124
in children, 16, 23-25
algorithm for, *25*
clinical interview, 16, *25*, *26*, 32-33
comorbid conditions, 33-41
externalizing conditions, 35-36, 36t
internalizing conditions, 36-40, 38t
learning/language disorders, 33-35
motor disorders/physical conditions, 40-41
other behavioral disorders, 35-40
substance-use disorders, 122-124, *123*
continuum and context of behaviors in, 29
criteria, 23, 24t
age and, 27t, 28
changes in, 18
core symptoms, 24t, 29
DSM criteria, *11*, 12, 18, 23, 28
functional impairment, importance of, 28, 31
hyperactivity/impulsivity dimension, 24t
inattention dimension, 24t
normative, lack of, 17
other criteria, 27-28
persistence of symptoms, 27t, 28
developmental level and, 23, 28
differential diagnosis, 28, 31, 32-33
history in, 32-33
individual variability and, 16
misdiagnosis/underdiagnosis, 19-20
neurologic exam, *25*, *26*
other medical conditions and, 28
physical exam, *25*, *26*, 32
rating scales, 30-32, 30t, 91-92, *134-145*
sources of information, 23-27, 27t
for adults, 25-26, 92
for children, 23-25
disagreements in, 26-27, 27t, 29
other than parents and teachers, 27t, 29
parents, 23-27
self reports, 16
subjectivness in, 16, 17-18
teachers, 23-27, 29
"subsyndromal" patients, 29-30
tests and assessments, 30-32
Diagnostic and Statistical Manual of Mental Disorders. See *DSM*.
Dietary supplements, 113-114
Diets for ADHD, 111-113
Feingold diet, 111-112
oligoantigenic (oligoallergenic, Few-Foods) diet, 112
sugar-restriction diet, 112-113

11

Dimethylaminoethanol, 115
Discipline/punishment, in behavior-modification training, 103, 104t, 105
Dopamine neurotransmitter systems, 16, 63
Dopamine transporter gene (DAT1), 15
Driving (motor vehicle), 52, 94
 accidents/violations, 20, 52, 120
 advice and cautions about, 125, 126t
Drug abuse/dependence. See *Substance-use disorders.*
Dry mouth
 α-adrenergic medications and, 90
 lisdexamfetamine and, 86
DSM (Diagnostic and Statistical Manual of Mental Disorders), *11*, 12
 ADHD criteria in different versions, *11*, 12, 18, 23, 24t, 28
 ADHD prevalence rates and, 18, *18*, 19
 comorbidity definition, 33
 depressive/manic episodes, criteria for, 38t
 DSM-IV
  ADHD criteria in, *11*, 12, 23, 24t, 28
  ADHD prevalence rates and, 18, *18*
 DSM for Primary Care Child and Adolescent Version, 29
 rating scales, 30-32, 30t, 32t
 substance abuse/dependence criteria, 126t-127t
 "subsyndromal" behaviors, 29
DuPaul Parent and Teacher Rating Scales, 30, 30t
Dyes, food, 111-112
Dyslexia, 33

ECGs (electrocardiograms)
 stimulant medications and, 79, 81
 tricyclic antidepressants and, 89
Education
 accommodations in, 54-55, 105-106, 109
 on ADHD, for patients and family, 47, 49, 55-56
 individual education plan (IEP), 106
 mainstreaming in, 106
EEG biofeedback, 115
Electrocardiograms (ECG), 79, 81, 89
Electroencephalogram (EEG), 31
Employment
 accommodations in, 54-55, 105-106, 109
 career choices, 54-55
Encepahlitis, influenza, 10
Essential fatty acids (EFAs), 113
Etiology of ADHD, 15-16
Evidence-based Psychotherapies for Children and Adolescents (Kazdin and Weisz, eds.), 100t
Executive function, 30, 122
Exercises and training, 115-116
Externalizing conditions, 35-36, 36t

Facts for Families, 57
Family. See also *Parents.*
education for, 47, 49
involvement in ADHD management, 45, 46-47
Family history
of ADHD, 15, 55
of bipolar disorder, 36-37
Family therapy, 99
Fatigue
α-adrenergic medications and, 90
major depression and, 38t
FDA-approved medications, 59-88, 66t.
See also *Medications for ADHD.*
Feedback
EEG biofeedback, 115
for patients (on ADHD treatment/progress), 46, 47-49, 107, 108t
Feingold diet, 111-112
Females, ADHD prevalence in, 12, 19
Fetal alcohol syndrome, 15, 41
Few-Foods diet, 112
Fire department, career in, 55
Focalin, Focalin XR. See *Dexmethylphenidate.*
Food additives, preservatives, and dyes, 111-112
Fragile X syndrome, 32, 41
Functional magnetic resonance imaging (fMRI), 16

Gender, ADHD prevalence and, 12, 19
Generalized anxiety disorder (GAD), 39
Genetic diseases mimicking ADHD symptoms, 32
Genetic factors in ADHD, 15, 55
GI constrictures, 71
Ginkgo biloba, 114
Growth potential (height), 61, 76
Guanfacine (Tenex), 89-90

Head injuries, 32, 41
Headache
amphetamines and, 81
history of, 75-76
methylphenidate and, 75-76
modafinil and, 91
Health care organizations, 45-46, 46t
Health questionnaires. See *Rating scales.*
Heart (cardiac) side effects, 78-79, 128t
Heart disorders
congenital, 78
family history of, 78
Height, 61, 76
monitoring, 61, 92
Helping the Noncompliant Child (Forehand and McMahon), 101t

11

Hepatotoxicity, atomoxetine and, 86
Herbal compounds, 114
Heritability, ADHD and, 15, 55
History of ADHD, 9-12
Hoffman, Heinrich, 9
Hyperactive child syndrome, *11*, 12
Hyperactivity
  criterion in ADHD diagnosis, 23, 24t, 27t
  persistence into adulthood, 20
  predominantly hyperactive/impulsive subtype of ADHD, 12, 24t, 28
  as secondary deficit in ADHD, 12
  "subsyndromal," 29
  withdrawal from substance use and, 124
Hypertension, 56, 78
Hypotension, 90

IDEA (Individuals with Disability Education Act), 105-106
IEP (individual education plan), 106
Imipramine (Tofranil), 89
Impulsivity
  criterion in ADHD diagnosis, 23, 24t
  withdrawal from substance use and, 124
Inattention
  criterion in ADHD diagnosis, 23, 24t
  predominantly inattentive subtype of ADHD, 12, 19, 24t, 27
  as primary deficit in ADHD, 12
  "subsyndromal," 29
  withdrawal from substance use and, 124
Incredible Years (*IY*) training, 101t
Individual education plan (IEP), 106
Individuals with Disability Education Act (IDEA), 105-106
Infections, ADHD and, 10, 15
Influenza epidemic (1917-1818), 10, *11*
Inheritance, ADHD and, 15, 55
Insomnia
  amphetamines and, 81, 86
  bupropion and, 90
  major depression and, 38t
  modafinil and, 91
Intelligence
  communication about, 49, 55-56
  standardized tests of, 34
Internalizing conditions, 36-40

Johnny Look-in-the-Air (Hoffman), 9-10

Kava hops, 114
Ketoconazole, 114
Klinefelter's syndrome, 32

Language assessment, 105-106
Language disorders, 33-35
Lead exposure, 15, 31, 32
Learning and language disorders, 32, 33-35, 122
  substance use disorder and, 122
Learning disabilities, 28, 94
Lemon balm, 114
Linoleic/linolenic acids, 113
Lisdexamfetamine (Vyvanse), 66t, 81-86. See also *Amphetamines.*
  abuse potential, reduced, 64, 81-83, 128
  dose, 64, 66t, 91
  duration of action, *80*, 83
  efficacy, 83-86, *84-85*, *87*
  as prodrug, 81-83
  side effects, 86
  tolerability, 86
  vs mixed amphetamine salts, 83, *84-85*
Listlessness, stimulant medications and, 76
Long-term outcomes of ADHD, 20-21

Magnetic resonance imaging (MRI), 16, 31
Mainstreaming, in schools, 106
Males, ADHD prevalence in, 12, 19
Management plan for ADHD, 46-49, *48*.
    See also *Treatment of ADHD.*
  for adolescents, 50-55, 53t, 62
  for adults, 55-57
  behavioral interventions in, 99-110
  form for, *48*
  goals in, 47
  patient/family involvement in, 45, 46-47, 62
  self-management support, 45, 46-47, 46t
Manic episodes, 36-37, 38t
Marijuana use/abuse, 119, 121
Marital relations, 20, 56
MBD. See *Minimal cerebral brain dysfunction/damage.*
Medications for ADHD, 59-97. See also *specific medications.*
  abuse potential, lower, 64, 81-83, 128
  for adults, 12, 13
  algorithms
    for preschool-age, *92*
    for primary school through adult, *93*
  alternative, 114-115
  career choice and, 55
  for comorbid conditions, timing of, 63
  consent of patient and, 50
  coverage needs, 94
  diversion of, 94, 125-128
    guidelines for avoidance and recognition of, 127-128, 128t
    red flags and precautions for, 128t

Medications for ADHD *(continued)*
efficacy, 13, 60-63
FDA-approved, 59-88, 66t
individual differences in response to, 74-75, 76, 80, 91
management of, 91-95
monitoring of, 91-94
non-FDA-approved, 88-91
α-adrenergic medications, 89-90
bupropion, 90
modafinil, 90-91
tricyclic antidepressants, 89
nonstimulant medications (atomoxetine), 86-88, *88*
selection of, 64, 91
stimulant medications, 59-88, 66t
age and, 60-61
amphetamines, 66t, 79-86
blood concentration over time, 59, *60*
cardiac side effects, 78-79
choice of, 64, 91
differences in, 63
dosing and pharmacokinetics, 66t, 76-78, *77*, 91
efficacy, 60-63, *61*
history of, 59
lisdexamfetamine, 66t, 81-86
methylphenidate, 65-79, 66t
misconceptions, 63-64
response rates, 60-61, *61*
safety, 61-62, 63
substance-use disorders and, 126t-127t
titration, 64-65, 91
substance abuse concerns and, 119
in substance-use disorders, 126t-127t
titration of, 64-65, 91, 92
Megavitamins, 113
Melatonin, 114
Meningitis, 15
Mental health specialists
links with, 46, 47
referral to, *92*, *93*
Mental retardation, 34
Metadate CD (methylphenidate), 66t, 69-70.
See also *Methylphenidate.*
dosing and pharmacokinetics, 66t, 77
duration of action, *77*
efficacy, 69-70, *70*
Methylin, Methylin ER (methylphenidate), 66t.
See also *Methylphenidate.*
Methylphenidate (MPH), *11*, 65-79, 66t
blood concentration over time, *60*
blood count, monitoring, 78

Methylphenidate (MPH) *(continued)*
contraindications, 71
controversy about, 13
dosing and pharmacokinetics, 64, 66t, 76-77, 91
dose response, *61*
duration of action, 65, 69, 77-78, *77*
Metadate CD, 69
OROS-MPH (Concerta), 71
Ritalin SR, 69
transdermal patch (Daytrana), 74-75
efficacy, 60-63, *61*, 65-75
dexmethylphenidate (Focalin), 73-74, *74*
Metadate CD, 69-70, *70*
methylphenidate patch (Daytrana), 74-75, *75*
OROS-MPH (Concerta), 71-72, *72*, *73*
Ritalin LA, 70-71, *71*
formulations, 65, 66t, 76-77
with lower abuse potential, 64
microbead technology, 69, 71, 73
osmotic pump, 71
transdermal patch, 64, 66t, 74-75
half-life, 65
in medication algorithms, *92*, *93*
response rates/response to second medication, 65-69, 67t, 68t
safety profiles, 63
seizures and, 63
selection of, 91
side effects, 75-76
cardiac, 78-79
vs dexamphetamine, 65, 67t, 68t
Microbead technology, 69, 71, 73
Minimal cerebral brain dysfunction/damage (MBD), 10-12, *11*, 13
Mixed amphetamine salts. See *Amphetamine salts, mixed.*
Modafinil (Provigil), 90-91
Molds, antifungal agents for, 114-115
Mood disorders, 28, 36-39, 38t, 63
Motor disorders/dysfunction, 31, 40-41
Motor vehicle accidents/violations, 20, 52, 120
advice and cautions about, 125, 126t
MPH. See *Methylphenidate.*
MRI (magnetic resonance imaging), 16, 31
Multi-Modal Therapy of ADHD (MTA) trial, 63
Multidimensional Anxiety Scale for Children, 35
Multiple sclerosis, 32
Myths about ADHD, 9-12

National Attention-Deficit Disorders Association, 56
National Guard, participation in, 55
National Institute for Mental Health (web site), 56
National Parent Information Network, 100t

11

National Resource Center for ADHD (web site), 57
Nausea, bupropion and, 90
Neurologic exam, *25*, *26*
Nicotine exposure, 15
Non-FDA-approved medications, 88-91.
  See also *Medications for ADHD.*
Nonstimulant medications, 86-88
Nootropic medications, 115
Norepinephrine neurotransmitter systems, 16, 63
  atomoxetine and, 86
  stimulant medications and, 63
  tricyclic antidepressants and, 89
Norpramin (desipramine), 89
Nortriptyline (Pamelor), 89
Nystatin, 114
NYU Child Study Center, 100t

Obsessive-compulsive disorder (OCD), 40
Obstructive sleep apnea, 32
ODD. See *Oppositional defiant disorder.*
Oligoantigenic (oligoallergenic) diet, 112
Omega-3 fatty acids, 113
1-2-3 Magic: Effective Discipline for Children (Phelan), 100t
Oppositional defiant disorder (ODD), 35-36, 36t
OROS-methylphenidate (Concerta), 66t, 71-72.
  See also *Methylphenidate.*
  abuse potential (reduced), 64, 128
  approval for adults, 72
  blood concentration over time, *60*
  contraindications, 71
  dosing and pharmacokinetics, 64, 66t, 77, 91
  duration of action, *77*
  efficacy, 71-72, *72*, *73*
Osmotic pump (OROS-methylphenidate), 71
Outcomes, long-term, 20-21
Overfocussing, stimulant medications and, 76, 80

Pamelor (nortriptyline), 89
PANDAS (pediatric autoimmune neuropsychiatric disorders
  associated with streptococcal infections), 40
Panic attacks, 39
Parent-Child Interaction Therapy (PCIT), 100-103, 101t-102t
Parent Global Perceptions questionnaire, 65
Parent Management Training Oregon Model (PMTO), 102t
Parenting the Strong-Willed Child (Forehand and Long), 100t
Parents. See also *Rating scales.*
  communication with teachers, 107
  disagreement with reports of, 17-18, 26-27, *27t*
  parent-training programs, 99-105, 101t-103t
    books and resources on, 100t

Parents, parent-training programs (continued)
elements of, 103-105, 104t
as source of information for diagnosis/monitoring, 17-18, 23-25, 92
Passionflower, 114
Patient
destigmatizing ADHD in communication with, 49, 55-56
education for, 47, 49, 55-56
feedback for, 46, 47-49, 107, 108t
involvement in management plan/process, 46-47, 50-51, 62
self-management, support for, 45, 46-47
support groups for, 56
Pediatric autoimmune neuropsychiatric disorders associated with streptococcal infections (PANDAS), 40
Pemoline, 59
Permanent Product Measure of Performance (PERMP), 83, *84-85*
PERMP (Permanent Product Measure of Performance), 83, *84-85*
Pervasive developmental disorders, 28, 32
Phobias, 39
Physical conditions, comorbid with ADHD, 41
Physical exam, *25*, *26*, 32
Piracetam, 115
Pittsburgh Side Effects-Rating Scale, *146-147*
Play therapy, 99
Police department, career in, 55
Positive attention and reinforcement, 103-105, 104t
Positive Parenting Program (Triple P), 102t-103t
Positron emission tomography, 16
Posttraumatic stress disorder (PTSD), 39
Prefrontal cortex, 16, 63
Premature birth, ADHD and, 15
Preservatives, food, 111-112
Prevalence of ADHD, 16-20, *18*, 119
difficulties in determining, 16-19
DSM changes and, 18, *18*
gender and, 12, 19
race/ethnicity and, 19
sampling and, 18-19
substance abuse disorders and, 119-120
variance in, 19
Prevalence of comorbid conditions, 33
Provigil (modafinil), 90-91
Psychoeducational counseling, 27t
Psychoeducational tests, 34
Psychosocial treatments, 99-110
adolescent and adult behavioral interventions, 107-109
communication/daily report card (DRC), 107, 108t
parent-training programs, 99-105, 100t, 101t-103t
school services, 105-107
Psychotic symptoms, stimulant medications and, 76, 80

Punishment, in behavior-modification training, 103, 104t, 105
Pycnogenol, 114

Questionnaires. See *Rating scales.*

Race/ethnicity, ADHD prevalence and, 19
Rating scales, 30-32, 30t, 32t, 91-92, *134-147*
  adult, for retrospective symptoms, 32
  Adult Self-Rating Scale (ASRS), 31-32
  Barkley version, 31
  Brown Adult ADD Scale, 32t
  Brown Adults Attention Disorder Scale (BAADS), 32
  communication and, 49
  for comorbid conditions, 35
  Conners Adolescent ADD Scale, 32t
  Conners Adolescent ADHD scale, 30t, 31
  Conners Adult ADD Scale, 32t
  Conners Adult ADHD Rating Scale (CAARS), 31
  Conners Teacher and Parent Rating Scales, Revised, 30, 30t
  core symptom monitoring with, 91-94
  in diagnosis, *25*, *26*, 91
  DSM-IV-based
    for adults, 31-32, 32t
    for children and adolescents, 30-31, 30t
  DuPaul Parent and Teacher Rating Scales, 30, 30t
  Parent Global Perceptions questionnaire, 65
  Pittsburgh Side Effects-Rating Scale, *146-147*
  SKAMP, 31
  SNAP-IV, 30, 30t, 31
  specific medication assessments with
    dexamphetamine, 65, 67t, 68t
    lisdexamphetamine, 83-86, *84-85*, *87*
    methylphenidate, 65, 67t, 68t, 69-75, *70*, *71*, *74*, *75*
    mixed amphetamine salts, 81, *82*
  Vanderbilt Parent-Assessment Scale, 30, 31, 92, *134-137*
  Vanderbilt Parent-Assessment Scale Follow-up, *138-139*
  Vanderbilt Teacher-Assessment, 30, 92, *140-143*
  Vanderbilt Teacher-Assessment Follow-up, *144-145*
Reading disabilities, 33-34
Rehabilitation Act (504), 105
Reinforcement, in behavior-modification training, 103-105, 104t
Resources
  ADHD web sites, 56-57
  on parent training, 100t
Rewards, in behavior-modification training, 103-105, 104t
Risk-taking behaviors, 52, 122
Ritalin, Ritalin LA, Ritalin SR, 59, 66t, 69. See also *Methylphenidate.*
  dosing and pharmacokinetics, 66t, 77
  duration of action, 69, *77*
  efficacy, 70-71, *71*

Rule violation
in conduct disorder, 37t
punishments for, 104t, 105

Salicylate compounds, avoiding, 111-112
Scales. See *Rating scales.*
Schizophrenia, childhood, 28
School services, 105-107. See also *Education.*
Screening for substance-use disorders, 122-124, *123*
Sedation
α-adrenergic medications and, 90
tricyclic antidepressants and, 89
Seizure disorders, 32, 63
Seizures
bupropion and, 90
dextroamphetamine and, 63
methylphenidate and, 63
Self-management, support for, 45, 46-47
Sensory integration, 115-116
Separation anxiety disorder (SAD), 39-40
Sickle cell anemia, 32
Single-photon emission computed tomography. See *SPECT.*
SKAMP rating scale, 31
lisdexamphetamine assessment with, 83, *84-85*
methylphenidate assessment with, 73-75, *74*, *75*
Sleep disorders, 32
modafinil for, 90
Sleep disturbance
amphetamines and, 81, 86
atomoxetine and, 86
clonidine as sleep aid, 90
history of, 75-76
methylphenidate and, 75-76
Smoking. See *Nicotine exposure.*
SNAP-IV rating scale, 30, 30t, 31
in evaluation of methylphenidate, 72
Social-skills training, 99, 106-107
Soft neurologic signs, 10, 31
Somnolence, atomoxetine and, 86
SPECT (single-photon emission computed tomography), 16, 31
Speech assessment, 105-106
Stevens-Johnson syndrome, 90
Still, George, 10, *11*
Stimulant medications, 59-88, 66t. See also *Medications for ADHD; specific medications.*
abuse potential, lower, 64
amphetamines, 66t, 79-86
cardiac side effects, 78-79, 128t
coverage needs/daily activities and, 94
dexmethylphenidate, 66t, 73-74

11

Stimulant medications *(continued)*
differences in, 63
diversion of, 94, 125-128
guidelines for avoidance and recognition of, 127-128, 128t
red flags and precautions for, 128t
dosing and pharmacokinetics, 66t, 76-78, *77*, 91
efficacy, 60-63, *61*
core symptoms and, 62, 91-94
of second medication after non-response to first, 60, 65-69, 67t, 68t
short-term vs long-term, 62-63
history of, 59
individual differences in response, 74-75, 76, 80
lisdexamfetamine, 66t, 81-86
in medication algorithms, *92*, *93*
methylphenidate, *11*, 65-79, 66t
response rates, 60-61, *61*
safety, 61-62, 63, 78-79
selection of, 64, 91
substance-use disorders and, 126t-127t
titration, 64-65, 92
Strattera (atomoxetine), 86-88, *92*
Strictures of the GI tract, 71
Students With Disabilities Office, registering with, 54-55
Substance abuse. See *Substance-use disorders.*
Substance-use disorders (SUDs), 62, 119-132
abuse of stimulant medications, 64
ADHD medications and, 126t-127t
algorithm for assessment and treatment, *123*
bipolar disorder and, 121
conduct disorder (CD) and, 36, 120, 121
counseling for, 109
diagnosis of ADHD in, 124
diversion of stimulant medications, 125-128
guidelines for avoidance and recognition of, 127-128, 128t
red flags and precautions for, 128t
DSM-IV criteria, 126t-127t
feigning of ADHD to get medications, 124
level of use/abuse, 126t-127t
overlap with ADHD, 20, 119-121
predictive factors for, 121-122
prevalence of, 119
coexisting with ADHD, 20, 119-120
prognosis for, ADHD and, 121-122
risk of, in adolescents, 52
screening and assessment, 122-124, *123*
treatment of, *123*, 124-125, 126t-127t
"Subsyndromal" patients, 29-30
Subtypes of ADHD, *11*, 12, 23, 27-28
combined types, 28
core symptoms of, 24t

Subtypes of ADHD *(continued)*
predominantly hyperactive/impulsive type, 12, 24t, 28
predominantly inattentive type, 12, 19, 24t, 27
Sudden cardiac death (SCD), 78, 79
Sugar-restriction diet, 112-113
Suicidal ideation, atomoxetine and, 86
Supplements, dietary, 113-114
Support groups, 56
Swallowing, difficulty with, 65, 73, 81, 83
Swanson, Kotin, Atkins, M-Flynn, and Pelham Department rating scale. See *SKAMP rating scale.*
Symptoms of ADHD
compensation for, 28, 45, 50, 94
continuing into adulthood, 9, 12, 20
core, 24t, 29
monitoring of, 91-94
duration of, diagnosis and, 27t, 28
mimicked by other conditions, 32

Teachers. See also *Rating scales.*
communication with parents, 107
disagreement with parents, 17-18, 26-27, 27t
feedback from, 47-49
involvement in management plan, 45
as source of information for diagnosis/monitoring, 17-18, 23-25, 92
Tenex (guanfacine), 89-90
Testing accommodations, 55, 105-106
Thyroid hormone, unresponsiveness to, 41
Tics and tic disorders, 40
amphetamines and, 80
methylphenidate and, 76
Timeline of ADHD history, *11*
Tobacco use, 119
Tofranil (imipramine), 89
Token system of rewards, 104-105
Tourette's disorder, 40. See also *Tics and tic disorders.*
Trauma
brain, ADHD and, 15-16
closed head injuries, 32, 41
Treatment of ADHD
alternative treatments, 111-118
alternative medications, 114-115
communicating with patient about, 116
dietary supplements, 113-114
diets, 111-113
exercises and training, 115-116
behavior modification, 99-105, 100t, 101t-103t, 107-109
chronic-illness approach, 45-57, 46t
community/health care resources, 45-46, 46t
feedback in, 47-49, 107, 108t

Treatment of ADHD *(continued)*
goals for, 47
management plan, 46-49, *48*. See also *Management plan for ADHD.*
for adolescents, 50-55, 53t
for adults, 55-57
medications, 59-97. See also *Medications for ADHD; and specific medications.*
alternative, 114-115
FDA-approved, 59-88, 66t
management of, 91-95
methylphenidate, 65-79
non-FDA-approved, 88-91
nonstimulant, 86-88
stimulant, 59-88, 66t
substance-use disorders and, 126t-127t
monitoring and follow-up, 46, 47, 91-94
psychosocial treatments, 99-110
adolescent and adult behavioral interventions, 107-109
communication/daily report card (DRC), 107, 108t
parent-training programs, 99-105, 100t, 101t-103t
school services, 105-107
self-management support, 45
written treatment plan, 47, *48*
Treatment of substance-use disorders, *123*, 124-125, 126t-127t
Tricyclic antidepressants, 59, 89
Triple P (Positive Parenting Program), 102t-103t
Tutoring, 99
Twin studies, 15

Valerian root, 114
Vanderbilt Rating Scales, 30-31, 92
Parent-Assessment Scale, 30, 31, *134-137*
Parent-Assessment Scale Follow-up, *138-139*
Teacher-Assessment, 30, *140-143*
Teacher-Assessment Follow-up, *144-145*
Vitamins
megavitamins, 113
vitamin C, deficiency of, 112
Vyvanse. See *Lisdexamfetamine.*

Web sites
ADHD, 56-57, 100t
parent training, 100t
rating scales, 30t, 32t
Wechsler Adult Intelligence Scale (WAIS), 34
Wechsler Intelligence Scale for Children, 4th Edition (WISC-IV), 34
Weight loss
amphetamines and, 81
major depression and, 38t
methylphenidate and, 75

Wellbutrin (bupropion), 90
Wender, Paul, 32
Whites (Caucasians), ADHD prevalence among, 19
Wilson's disease, 32
Woodcock Johnson III Test of Achievement, Revised, 34
Work. See *Employment.*

Yeast, eliminating from diet, 114-115
Youth Forum, 35

Zinc supplements, 114

11